Lauren Kaplan

People Living with HIV in the USA and Germany

A Comparative Study of Biographical Experiences of Chronic Illness

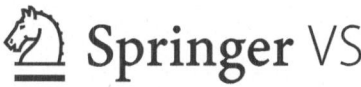 Springer VS

Lauren Kaplan
Oxford, United Kingdom

Dissertation Goethe University Frankfurt am Main, 2013

D 30

ISBN 978-3-658-05266-9   ISBN 978-3-658-05267-6 (eBook)
DOI 10.1007/978-3-658-05267-6

The Deutsche Nationalbibliothek lists this publication in the Deutsche Nationalbibliografie;
detailed bibliographic data are available in the Internet at http://dnb.d-nb.de.

Library of Congress Control Number: 2014933522

Springer VS
© Springer Fachmedien Wiesbaden 2014

Printed on acid-free paper

Springer VS is a brand of Springer DE.
Springer DE is part of Springer Science+Business Media.
www.springer-vs.de

People Living with HIV in the USA and Germany

Acknowledgments

This project was a collaborative effort facilitated by the support and guidance of an international and multidisciplinary academic exchange.

I would like to express my deepest appreciation for the invaluable guidance and support of Professor Lena Inowlocki, who served as the primary supervisor of my doctoral work at Goethe Univesity. With the support of Professor Lena Inowlocki, my work in Frankfurt was made possible and has truly inspired and fostered my personal and professional development. I would also like to thank Professor Heino Stöver and Professor Heidemarie Kremer for their contributions as members of my dissertation committee and for their advice and commentary, which helped to improve this research project. I also express my deep appreciation to Professor Gail Ironson, whose parent research project in Miami provided invaluable data that allowed for a comparative study. The additional research of Professor Gail Ironson and Professor Heidemarie Kremer in Miami helped to make this comparative study possible.

This work was made possible by collaborative efforts involving the University of Applied Sciences, Frankfurt, Goethe University, and the University of Miami. This research was facilitated by an Innovation Fund from the University of Applied Sciences to facilitate transnational migration research. These funds provided valuable financial support for this project.

Importantly, I would like to thank the physicians and staff at the University Clinic and the Helping Hand project, which was supported by the Deutsche AIDS Hilfe, for their support. I also express my sincere gratitude to those who shared their stories and made this research possible. I hope that while your identities are kept anonymous you will feel that this project contributes to a better understanding of the life conditions of people living with HIV/AIDS.

I would also like to thank my professors and advisors over the years who have supported my decision to leave the United States and to engage in international research.

This research would not have been possible without the invaluable guidance and support of my family. I would like to convey my deepest gratitude to my mother Judy Kaplan for her ongoing love and support. I would also like to thank my uncle Charles Kaplan for his guidance, encouragement, and belief in my potential. I would also like to thank my closest friends who have supported my efforts over the years with understanding, an unwavering belief in my potential, and love.

Lauren Michelle Kaplan

Table of Contents

Preface

The purpose of this book is to illuminate the life experiences of people living with HIV. Challenges embedded in social policy such as access, cost, and availability of quality medical care and immigration policies which can restrict the freedom of people to travel, work, and live in different nations and regions are a focus of this book. Stigma and discrimination and existential struggles of identity, meaning, and reality are another major focus of this work. While these challenges are made visible in the examination of the biographical experiences of people living with HIV, they can also be considered as important issues for human rights more generally. In the context of a global recession and increasing social, cultural, and economic international interdependence, comparative transnational studies are of an ever growing importance to our understanding of what policies and conditions are supportive of health and promoting the development of human potential.

People living with HIV suffer from an infectious disease which they can contract in ways through which contrary to popular opinion, they are not to blame. It is the author's imperative that people with illnesses such as HIV and other chronic illnesses such as cancer not be stigmatized or discriminated against in our contemporary global society. The challenges of negotiating a chronic illness are vast, and stigma can render such experiences especially problematic for those suffering from chronic illness. Therefore, the stories of interviewees in this book were selected not only for their substantive theoretical content but also to challenge prevailing negative stereotypes of HIV. Powerful stories of people living with HIV from a range of backgrounds were examined to emphasize the important fact that HIV is something that can happen to us all. Images of drug addiction and sexual responsibility have plagued the HIV-positive community. Such images are linked to risky behaviors which can lead to infection, but these do not define all people living with HIV. Furthermore, even for those with histories of drug use or sexual risk taking we must be reminded of our own sexual experiences and the potential for people to trust others to not use protection due to feelings of familiarity, love, and infatuation. Importantly, while injection drug use is a risk factor for the transmission of infectious diseases, having a history of drug use does not justify forsaking other's human dignity and rights and blaming and marginalizing those with such histories.

Human experience can be seen as a progression of our personal histories shaped in the context of broader social and economic historical context. Within each of our lives there is the potential for suffering, destruction, and for growth and transformation. Such potentialities highlight the fluid nature of our own existence and the important realization that our pasts, presents, and futures can unravel in unanticipated ways. HIV can be one of many unanticipated events in people's life stories. Moving away from blaming those suffering from chronic illness and moving towards a more nuanced, open, and compassionate under-standing of human experience is essential to the protection of human rights and dignity. An important goal of the present work is to facilitate such an under-standing.

Also important is that in the experience of HIV, aspects of social reality that otherwise may be hidden from our awareness our brought to the center stage. Issues in the negotiation of social interaction, threats to identity and mortality, and epistemological debates of the nature of truth, reality, and illusion are illuminated in the stories of people living with HIV with a vividness and urgency we may otherwise not encounter. Thus, this analysis is intended not only for the sociology student, scholar, or researcher, but for a broader audience of those concerned with human rights and the conditions and policies which govern their lives. It is the hope of the author that this work will help to facilitate a greater understanding of the lives of people with HIV, reduce stigmatizing views of those suffering from illness, and enhance an understanding of social reality both within and beyond the realm of HIV.

By engaging in a transnational comparison, we are better able to identify areas of strength and of weakness in domestic U.S. policy as compared to social policies in Germany. We also are able to understand how experiences of people are conditioned by their personal and collective histories and the broader social and economic context of their countries of residence. The areas of both conver-gence and similarity in experience, and of difference and departure in the lives of people living in Miami, the United States and Frankfurt, Germany, allow for an examination of how chronic illness can be understood by actors in distinct cultural contexts.

This book is organized in the following manner. First, a discussion of the re-gional and national contexts in Miami and Frankfurt, the concept of a trajectory of suffering, and other key concepts such as stigma in their relation to HIV are discussed. Next, the methodology used to examine these biographies is presented. The biographical analysis utilized here grew in a transnational exchange between the U.S. and Germany. There is a deep interrelation between theory, methodology, and findings. Therefore, an understanding of the methodological approach used in this work frames the analysis in theoretical context.

Next, the findings are presented. These findings are divided into the following parts: (1) conditional aspects of the emergence of a trajectory of suffering; (2) biographical process structures; (3) theoretical aspects of negotiating HIV, and (4) structural aspects of negotiating HIV. Finally, the discussion summarizes key findings, unanticipated phenomena, policy implications, limitations, strengths, and directions for future research.

1   Introduction

1.1   Biography and HIV as a Trajectory of Suffering

The purpose of this study was to examine how people living with HIV/AIDS (henceforth referred to as PLWHA) experience their illness and negotiate constraints such as stigma and other forms of marginalization, such as racism and poverty, and work to overcome trajectories of suffering. A major aim of my research was to examine how HIV was coped with and negotiated. Accordingly, I utilized a biographical approach in this comparative study of interviews with people living with HIV in Frankfurt, Germany and in Miami, Florida, the United States of America. Since the advent of effective treatment, HIV has been redefined from a "death sentence" to a "chronic illness" (Antiretroviral Therapy Cohort Collaboration 2008). HIV is of particular interest and relevancy to the biographical research tradition due to its initial disruptive character upon diagnosis which requires people to integrate HIV into their biographies, confront issues of mortality and self, and to continuously contend with its enduring stigma. HIV presents a formidable challenge as people with HIV must confront issues relating to not only their health, but also of morality, conceptions of sin, and sexuality (UNAIDS 2005).

Importantly, the health care system in the United States has recently begun a major transformation with the implementation of the Affordable Care Act (ACA). This policy shift is so controversial that members of the Tea Party, a conservative Republican political party, actively shut down the American government in their negotiations with President Barack Obama. The recent governmental shutdown and ongoing controversy surrounding health care policy suggests there is a need for researchers to examine health care policy in order to provide governmental agencies with an evidence-based approach to the implementation and ongoing evaluation of health care policy.

Germany provides a useful comparison to the American health care system. In this work, I utilize a patient-centered approach to understanding the experiences of people living with HIV/AIDS both in the health care system and in the broader context of their personal histories and the cultural context in which they are embedded.

Furthermore, with increasing global interdependence, the importance of health care is heightened in the context of migration. The United Nations has expressed a deep concern for the welfare of asylum seekers who often must live in overcrowded housing and have limited access to employment opportunities and health care (UN 2012). Access to health care for asylum seekers in Europe has been problematic, as access to health care is often limited to emergency care and as migrants can face legal and practical barriers to care (Norredam et al. 2005). Recently, because of military conflict in the Middle East, there has been a wave of migration to Europe. The political conflicts in nations such as Syria and Libya have had widespread global consequences greatly increasing the numbers of migrants to Europe. As of October 2013, it has been reported that over 32,000 migrants from the Middle East and Africa immigrated to Italy and Malta (Reuters 2013).

This recent wave of migration has sparked debates between the Southern and Northern European Union States as nations such as Italy called for support in the "burden sharing" of asylum seekers and financial resources. Reports suggest that political debates and rising anti-immigration attitudes delayed assistance to migrants and that this delay in support has coincided with the deaths of many migrants (Reuters 2013). Migration experiences can be further problematized by HIV and, through the use of narrative interviews, the issues of asylum-seeking in Germany emerged as a critical part of biography. The importance of access to specialized care and the context of medication adherence in group housing with limited privacy emerged in this study and will be further discussed in later chapters.

An examination of both the strengths and limitations in different policies allows for an interchange between policies with the potential for improvement. For example, in Germany, the importance of mainstreaming or the integration of HIV into multiple policy sectors has been a great advance in combating the HIV epidemic (Deutsche Gesellschaft für Internationale Zusammenarbeit (GIZ) GmbH 2012). The successful implementation of HIV policy into workplace programs for families in low- and middle-income countries has been accomplished through the work of Germany's Federal ministry for Economic Cooperation and Development (BMZ) (GIZ 2012). The close political ties between Germany and their partners in Sub-Saharan Africa have been paralleled by economic cooperation and intensive policy work to combat the HIV epidemic in Africa. The successful implementation of HIV programs into policies within multiple sectors suggests that in order to facilitate effective HIV policy, research done in comparative context can inform the work of various nation's efforts to improve health locally and globally.

Therefore, in the context of the contemporary global problems and events related to HIV, health care policy change, and migration in Europe, this comparative study contributes to an increased understanding of challenges faced by people living with HIV/AIDS. By engaging in a biographical analysis centered on patient experiences from a range of social backgrounds grounded in transnational comparative context, valuable insights were gained into the context of health care and migration issues that require an integrated, rigorous, and ongoing evidence-based approach to social policy.

1.2 Research Questions

Prior to initiating the analysis, stigma and social support were concepts of central interest. However, in order to gain a deeper understanding of interviewee's life experiences, open-ended narrative interviews were utilized. As the narrative interviews completed in Frankfurt, Germany were analyzed using the biographical approach, unanticipated phenomena and important biographical processes emerged, which informed the analysis of the Miami interviews. Throughout this process, research questions and analysis shared a dynamic interplay and my original questions became more open and flexible to accommodate new insights generated by the analysis. The research questions of this study are:

(1) How do people with HIV/AIDS (PLWHA) experience their illness?
(2) In which ways does HIV become a part of one's biography?
(3) Under what conditions can trajectories of suffering be overcome and what types of biographical action schemes are related to coping with HIV?

Because HIV can present both an immediate mortality threat upon diagnosis and yet can be lived with over time as a chronic illness, understanding how HIV is integrated into existing frames of reference and meaning can clarify how the initial existential threat of HIV can be negotiated into one's biography. HIV diagnosis can be stressful, shocking, and charged with emotional upset and feelings of being thrown into a new life against one's will (Kelly et al. 1998; Safren et al. 2003). Therefore, I examine HIV using a biographical perspective and examine HIV as an experience involving biographical processes. Gerhard Riemann and Fritz Schütze's (Riemann and Schütze 1991) conceptualization of a trajectory of suffering guided the analysis of how HIV was coped with over time. They defined trajectory of suffering as:

"A generalized concept of trajectory as a central category denoting *disorderly social processes and processes of suffering,* a category that makes it possible to identify, reconstruct and understand phenomena [...] We have in mind structural processes structured by conditional chains of events that one cannot avoid without high costs, constant breaks of expectations, and a growing and irritating sense of loss of control over one's life circumstances. One feels that one is driven, that one can only react to 'outer forces' that one does not understand anymore. There are conditions or seeds for the emergence of a trajectory (first just as potential), a step of crossing from the sphere of intentional action to the sphere of just reacting, different phases a trajectory is passing through, and, of course, there are ways out, too." (p. 377)

Importantly, biographical processes can overlap, and trajectories of suffering can be overcome. The experience of trajectory from its inception to its unfolding and the mastery of life circumstances were a major focus of this analysis. Therefore, I also examined the "ways out" of trajectory and focused on biographical action schemes. Biographical action schemes involve purposeful action aimed at the achievement of regaining control over one's life (Schütze 1981; 2007). This emphasized biographical action schemes as a means of understanding how participants became aware of their agency and enacted their agency in the working world (Schütz 1962). Agency must be enacted in the working world in order to initiate change in personal and collective social space. The importance of HIV disclosure in situating action out of the realms of phantasm and into the working world emerged as important to action. The enactment of agency can be fundamentally shaped by biography and socio-historical context. Therefore, a comparison of narratives created in a diverse sample was especially useful in the examination of agency. Biographical analysis is a useful approach that facilitated an analysis of agency by focusing on biographical action schemes. The conceptualization of trajectory as a structural process as involving "inner events" related to changes in personal identity allowed the interplay between individual experience and social structural conditions to be analyzed (Riemann and Schütze 1991, p. 339). The biographical constructions of people living with HIV were examined in the current study while also focusing on the social and historical context within which their personal biographies were embedded.

Identity and sense of belonging emerged in both samples as multidimensional concepts that were intimately tied to personal history. By focusing on identity, potentialities and constraints for overcoming the stigmatized social status of HIV, and even turning a marginalized position into an activist identity were identified. Qualitative researchers have used the term identity and emphasized the importance of the self in relation to suffering (Charmaz 1999) and have identified biographical processes for example the metamorphosis of identity to understand biography (Riemann and Schütze 1991). Importantly, in my analysis conceptions of the self and struggles with identity emerged as central to biographical experiences. Biographical researchers have also focused on the concept of mental space and the importance of the construction of a sense of belonging by relating to collective frames of reference and meaning in orienting the self and biographical development (Schütze et al. 2010). Accordingly, in my analysis, interviewees emphasized collective frames of reference in relation to their social positions and HIV status. The intersectionality of social positions and meanings ascribed to collective group membership emerged as important in processes related to the development of a sense of belonging. Accordingly, when describing the characteristics of a trajectory of suffering Riemann and Schütze (1991) described:

> "The overwhelming and long-lasting process of suffering gives the person the chance of systematic reflection, of finding a deep relationship to her- or himself and to the world and to significant others, and of mobilizing biographical work and creativity. This can be followed by well-organized biographical action schemes for controlling the dynamics of disorder and by the exploration and development of hirtherto unseen personal capabilities, that is, by a creative metamorphosis of the state of biographical identity." (p. 343 f.)

Therefore, the use of the term identity was not considered to be antithetical to the biographical approach. Rather, identity emerged as a temporally and culturally based concept integral to personal growth and development and was interrelated with issues related to action, empowerment, and integrating HIV into one's biography. Creativity, innovation, and the integration of HIV status into one's self-concept were emergent phenomenon that became a major focus of this study.

Importantly, the term identity was conceptualized as fluid and not static in this study. Identity was seen as a dynamic concept, involving a changing sense of belonging to different social statuses that was interrelated with personal and collective history, other life experiences, and concepts such as stigma. A sense of belonging has been defined in prior research "as the experience of personal involvement in a system or environment so that persons feel themselves to be an integral part of that system or environment" (Hagerty et al. 1992) and as a "sense of personal involvement in a social system so that persons feel themselves to be an indispensable and integral part of the system" (Anant 1966, p. 21). According to Hagerty and colleagues (1992), such systems can be organizations or relationships and therefore can involve social groups sharing particular social statuses, such as the status of being HIV-positive, gender, or sexual orientation. Sense of belonging involves both the feeling that one's involvement is valued and accepted and that one's characteristics fit with the social group (Hagerty et al. 1992). Sense of belonging is related to other concepts such as social support, feeling loved versus feeling alienated and isolated, and is related to identity and group membership (Hagerty et al. 1992). The interplay between sense of belonging, group identification, identity, and stigma were critical aspects of biological adjustment to living with HIV in interviewee's narratives. Specifically, these emerged as important concepts in the process of acceptance of HIV status and of coming to terms with illness.

Stigma was conceptualized as a process-based concept which involved more than a definition of a mark that is "deeply discrediting" (Goffman 1963). Stigma can involve numerous processes, such as processes in: identity, group identification, access to resources (economic and social), disclosure, and fear of identification. Prior research on stigma emphasizes the importance of focusing on power dynamics when analyzing stigma and of analyzing stigma as a process rather than as a static concept (Parker and Aggleton 2003; Link and Phelan 2001). Access to a collective identity can be a means to power. Having access to a collective identity in a positive, supportive context can help to transform stigmatized, marginalized self-concepts into empowered, activist identities or "project identities" (Castells 1997; Parker and Aggleton 2003).

By accessing and redefining collective identity from a marginalized group to an active, empowered group, collective identity of HIV can be transformed into a "project identity" (Castells 1997). Project identities involve the construction of a new identity that redefines a group's position in society and by transforming itself also aims to change the overall social structure (Castells 1997). By adopting a project identity, members can be empowered to initiate social change. Participation and membership in a community of mutual respect and support can provide access to power, contributing to empowerment, and helping people who are stigmatized to mobilize and spread awareness and understanding of their condition. Therefore, the concept of identity was important in understanding the meaning of taking part in "Helping Hand" an on-site support group. The Helping Hand support group is discussed in more detail in the description of the research setting in Frankfurt, Germany.

Drawing on Anselm Strauss (Strauss 1993) and his discussion of biographical work and processes in his seminal work "Permutations of Social Action," this analysis demonstrates that Strauss' formulation of processes central to biographical work were involved in participants' descriptions of their narratives. Strauss maintained that work is tied to all action and that all action may be conceptualized as a form of work. PLWHA are faced with a multitude of challenges and thus an analysis of HIV using a biographical perspective allows us to delve deeper into biographical processes and their relation to coping. Corbin and Strauss (1988) described the processes in biographical work as:

> "Four separate but overlapping *biographical processes*. Though analytically different, each process occurs simultaneously and feeds directly into the others. The processes are (1) *Contextualizing* (incorporating the [course of illness] into biography, (2) *coming to terms* (arriving at some degree of understanding and acceptance of the biological consequences of actual or potential failed performances), (3) *reconstituting identity* (reintegrating identity into a new conceptualization of wholeness around the limitations in performance), and (4) *recasting biography* (giving new directions to biography). Each of these processes evolves over time…[I]t is important to recognize analytically that [each of these processes] rests inevitably on the *biographical work* entailed in it." (p. 68 f.)

Therefore, coping with HIV was examined using this conceptualization of coping as involving biographical processes as they were intertwined with contextual experiences as discussed by participants.

1.3   HIV as Life-Changing

Anselm Strauss' (Stsrauss 1997) discussion of transformations of identity and turning points as the awareness that "I am not the same as I was, as I used to be" and involving misalignment or "surprise, shock, chagrin, tension, bafflement, self-questioning -- and also the need to try out the new self, to explore and validate the new and often exciting or frightening conceptions" highlights the importance of understanding life experiences such as HIV as a turning point with the potential for fundamental challenges and changes in life stories (Strauss 1997, p. 95). Prior research indicates that HIV can be a major life-changing event (Kremer et al. 2009). According to Kremer et al. (2009), HIV can serve as a positive or negative life-changing event with corresponding changes in behavior, self-view, worldview, and spirituality. Furthermore, they found that even when HIV was experienced as a negative turning point, a secondary positive turning point often occurred. They described two exceptional cases, one exemplifying a negative turning point and the other of HIV as a positive turning point. HIV as a negative turning point was described by participants in a manner consistent with the conceptualization of HIV as a trajectory of suffering. Interestingly, HIV as a positive turning point was discussed by participants in a manner fitting a biographical action scheme where they felt empowered to take action and to improve their own lives and even the lives of others.

Other studies suggest that people can experience post-traumatic growth or perceive positive changes since HIV diagnosis, which has also been referred to as "thriving" (O'Leary and Ickovics 1995; Siegel and Schrimshaw 2000; Milam 2006; Kremer and Ironson 2009). The concept of thriving has also been recognized in sociological research as being rooted in social positions and history (Blankenship 1998). This suggests that a biographical analysis was appropriate to further assess the role of HIV as a life-changing event that can involve numerous biographical processes as it is experienced in the context of personal biography and social context.

With the advent of highly active retroviral therapy (HAART) medication regimens, HIV has been transformed from a death sentence to a chronic illness (Scandlyn 2000; Siegel and Krauss 1991). This major shift in the definition of the meaning of having HIV as being transformed into a chronic illness that can be negotiated with over time highlights the importance of understanding how people negotiate their HIV condition in their everyday lives and work to incorporate their HIV diagnosis into their pre-existing social positions and their corresponding senses of belonging and self-views rooted in their biographies and social context. Indeed, Kremer et al. (2009) found that only 37 percent of their sample reported that HIV was a key turning point in their lives suggesting that HIV, while life-changing, should be examined in the context of personal experience and biography and not in a social vacuum. Researchers have suggested that a biographical approach to the study of coping with HIV is an important avenue for generating knowledge of HIV (Siegel and Krauss 1991).

Researchers have applied a biographical approach to understanding the lives of PLWHA and have found that people do work to reconstruct their identities in response to HIV diagnosis (Carricaburu and Pierret 1995). Biographical reconstruction has been argued to involve the construction of an identity that integrates HIV into biography and often reinforces aspects of identity prior to HIV diagnosis (Carricaburu and Pierret 1995). Notably, Pierret (2001) found that PLWHA often distinguish between their lives before and after HIV diagnosis thus incorporating a temporal dimension to their understanding of illness. Interestingly, as HIV became redefined from an initial death sentence to a chronic illness, research demonstrates that PLWHA wrestled with the question of why they were still alive (Pierret 2001). Existential struggles with mortality thus were not removed from the experiences of PLWHA even after the advent of effective HIV treatment.

Furthermore, Ciambrone (2001) in a study of HIV-positive women found that HIV should be considered in the broader context of women's lives. Ciambrone

(2001) found that the relative negative impact of HIV was dependent on other life experiences such as domestic violence, drug use, and separation from their children; and these life experiences were often discussed as more problematic than their HIV infection. The perception that HIV was not the main cause of biographical disruption in these women's lives was contextualized by whether or not they had access to social support, their racial/ethnic backgrounds, and drug use. In another biographical analysis of women with HIV/AIDS in Africa, Burchardt (2010) found that these women had to develop strategies of action to cope with the ontological uncertainty that their HIV diagnosis initiated in their lives. Burchardt (2010) emphasized the relationships between biographical context and action strategies and their relation to personal transformation, the search for normality, and social support. These action strategies were enabled and constrained in the context of religious discourse and AIDS activism (Burchardt 2010).

These biographical studies highlight the embededdness of life experience, the deep interrelation between life experiences, and the contextual conditions in which these experiences occur. Overall, prior research suggests that chronic illness can be a biographical disruption, upsetting notions of the self, the body, mortality, social relationships, and normality (Bury 1982; Burchardt 2010; Ciambrone 2001; Carricaburu and Pierret 1995; Charmaz 1983; 1995; Wilson 2007). Chronic illness can entail a deep suffering related to the self and is rooted in moral discourse (Charmaz 1999). Charmaz (1995) argued that the openness of others to hear the stories of those suffering can be affected by moral sentiments linked to the type of illness. This moral dimension can be especially problematic for PLWHA due to drug use and sexual behavior as commonly known causes of infection. These studies suggest that HIV can present an existential suffering that should be examined in the context of personal and collective biographies. PLWHA can experience a multitude of challenges and these are discussed below.

1.4 HIV and Stressful Life Conditions

Approximately 33 million people were living with Human Immunodeficiency Virus (HIV) in 2008, and AIDS has been identified as a cause of an estimated 25 million deaths worldwide (UNAIDS 2009; 2008). Estimates suggest that the extent of this epidemic has been underestimated and report that 40% more people than previously estimated became infected with HIV in 2006 (Hall et al. 2008). In addition, many PLWHA live in poverty, increasing their vulnerability to HIV/

AIDS (United Nations 2005). Living in a context of socioeconomic disadvantage can worsen the life conditions of those living with HIV. Specifically, research demonstrates that socioeconomic disadvantage can heighten levels of stress and decrease psychological resources such as social support, which can in turn lead to more adverse mental and physical health outcomes (Aneshensel 1992; Turner et al. 1995). Prior research indicates that stress can affect disease progression among PLWHA (Ironson et al. 2005; Leserman et al. 2000; 2002). Coping interventions among people living with HIV have been found to increase immune functioning and to reduce levels of anxiety and stress (Antoni et al. 2000). Research also suggests that social structural factors such as housing and poverty are associated with disease progression (Milloy et al. 2012). Furthermore, personality and physiological characteristics can interact with social context in their relationship to immune functioning (Capitanio et al. 2008). Importantly, stigma has been found to mediate the relationships between AIDS orphanhood and mental health outcomes such as psychological distress (Cluver et al. 2008). This suggests that the stigma of HIV can proliferate to family members and communities and demonstrates the impact that stigma can have on health and social functioning.

This emphasizes the importance of adopting a biopsychosocial model of health and engaging in interdisciplinary work informed by sociological approaches to understand HIV as a biographical experience. Biographical analysis allows for an examination of individual and social structural phenomena as interrelated and as mechanisms through which people can construct social reality. Biographical illness experience can have biological consequences for health and biographical research could inform future research on the interconnections between broader social conditions and personal experience. Specifically, the discovery of the meaning of illness and social positionality, as it occurs within the context of personal history and biography incumbents' broader social and economic life conditions, can help to unearth the processes linking the experience of illness, health behaviors, and health outcomes. For example, in my analysis, internal processes of denial were related to engaging in nondisclosure and unprotected sex and to a broader context of historical racism. Also, beliefs about the nature of medicine were related to participants' approaches to their medical treatment and were deeply embedded in their life histories. Interestingly, transformative processes such as resolving spiritual struggle emerged as important to the overcoming of drug addiction, which can affect health trajectories and utilization of care.

The World Health Organization's (1948) definition of health as complete physical, mental, and social well-being and not merely the absence of disease highlights the importance of the development and utilization of social resources (e.g. social networks and support), and material resources (e.g. financial security and medical care) in personal growth and development in the face of HIV. Personal growth and empowerment can be related to the biographical processes of action and metamorphosis of identity and to the development of sense of control, inspiration, and creative production. Resources can be conceptualized as factors that could be material (e.g., income and employment) or psychosocial (e.g., social support) and can serve to mitigate the negative impact of stressors on well-being. Resources can include social capital, psychosocial resources such as self-esteem, and economic resources. Pierre Bourdieu defined social capital as "the aggregate of the actual or potential resources which are linked to possession of a durable network of more or less institutionalized relationships of mutual acquaintance or recognition" (Bourdieu 1985, p. 248). Social networks and social capital can help to reduce stress, and prior research indicates that social resources are related to thriving (Blankenship 1998; Gächter et al. 2009; Massey et al. 1998). However, due to the stigmatized nature of HIV, people can prefer to live in secret with HIV, preventing their access to valuable social relationships and their corresponding resources.

Both initial HIV diagnosis and living with HIV as a chronic condition can be stressors. Stressors have been defined as "experiential circumstances that give rise to stress" and include life events (e.g. death of loved one) and chronic stressors (stressors which are enduring over time such as persistent poverty) (Pearlin 1989, p. 243). Because a major aim of this study was to understand how people, when faced with the existential crisis of life with HIV, work to succeed and to live meaningful and fulfilling lives, the roles of resources were analyzed as they emerged in the interviews. Social support and resources, agency, and social context were assessed in order to understand how people with HIV regained control over their lives. Social support and self-esteem have also been found to be related to posttraumatic growth or thriving and social positions rooted in race/ethnicity and gender also have been linked to thriving (Abraído-Lanza et al. 1998; Blankenship 1998; O'Leary 1998). An understanding of the processes involved in both the negative experience of stigma in tandem with coping and the conditions under which these processes unfold was a central aim of this analysis. Therefore, related issues of identity, adjustment to new social groups, and the negotiation of multiple social worlds such as intimate relationships, occupational careers, family relations, and importantly the interplay between the HIV-negative and HIV-positive social worlds are discussed. Biographical action schemes were therefore useful analytical concepts in this process.

A substantial number of those living with HIV can experience violent victimization, discrimination, social exclusion, engage in substance use and risky sexual behavior, and lose faith in themselves, society, and the spiritual (Bing et al. 2001; Michels et al. 2007; Kremer et al. 2009). Yet, despite "hitting rock bottom," many people living with HIV can manage to significantly change their lives and to improve their quality of life and social relationships. Siegel and Schrimshaw (2000) found in their study of women living with HIV that a majority of these women reported stress-related growth or thriving in response to HIV. These women reported positive changes in their health behaviors, spirituality, interpersonal relationships, self-view, value of life, and career goals. Thriving has been defined as "the ability to go beyond the original level of psychosocial functioning, to grow vigorously, to flourish" (O'Leary 1998, p. 429). Blankenship (1998) emphasized the applicability of a sociological perspective on thriving and urged future sociological research to focus on thriving. Massey and colleagues (Massey et al. 1998) emphasized the importance of using qualitative methodology when examining and conceptualizing thriving as a process rooted in personal and social history. They further argued that using qualitative methodology to examine thriving allows for an examination of context and of thriving as a process without imposing values a priori in the research process and asked:

> "How can researchers take seriously individuals' subjective experiences and also allow room for the powerful social, cultural, and political contexts within which these experiences occur? That is, how can we celebrate an individual's accomplishments and well-being in adverse situations without either blaming those whose lives show less cause for celebration, or dropping the critique of the contextual structures that promote the adversity? [and] How do we recognize that there may indeed be moments in which an individual in an adverse situation experiences joy, the successful completion of a meaningful piece of work, a sense of physical vigorousness, or other signs of thriving, but that there are also moments, in that very same life, absent of these desirable states?" (Massey et al. 1998, p. 338)

A biographical analysis can help to provide answers to these questions. As Massey and colleagues argue, by not restricting an analysis to a-priori variables of interest, researchers can identify structural factors that are theoretically relevant within participants' life stories. This process of discovery can facilitate theoretical development and the identification of important factors that can interact with experiences of adversity and thriving (Massey et al. 1998).

Indeed, unanticipated factors and processes emerged in the current study highlighting the usefulness of a biographical approach when examining thriving or biographical adjustment to HIV. Importantly, thriving can be a process and therefore is well-suited to a qualitative approach focusing on biography. Narratives allow us to examine trajectories of agency as ongoing processes that intersect with other biographical processes. These trajectories are grounded in the context of personal history and involve continued decision-making and biographical work. This provides us with an opportunity to engage in an analysis of the negotiation of stressors and challenges that is not framed in a static atheoretical framework. Instead, we are granted access to the temporal and contextual dimensions of theoretical concepts as they develop over time in biographical experience. This allows for a more process-oriented understanding and can stimulate theoretical developments in the production of knowledge (Massey et al. 1998).

Biographical processes involved in thriving in the face of adversity, specifically those related to action, can be of great import to the sociological study of stress, coping, and health. These processes were a major focus of this study. Survival, recovery, and thriving have been distinguished as distinct responses to hardship (O'Leary and Ickovics 1995). Thriving has been conceptualized as developing in an interactive and transformative process in coping with challenge (O'Leary, 1998, p. 429). By focusing on biographical experience, meaning making, and processes of suffering, transformation, and action a more nuanced understanding of thriving can be developed.

In addition, Pearlin and colleagues (Pearlin et al. 2005) applied a life course perspective to examine how and why those in disadvantaged social positions experience health disparities, such as higher levels of morbidity and mortality. They discussed three processes that can link stress to health outcomes. These included: status and status attainment, early life experiences and later life outcomes, and stress proliferation throughout the life course. These processes can be examined using narrative interviews. Pearlin et al. (2005) also focused on how educational deficits can lead to occupational disadvantage, which is linked with economic strains, and how life circumstances can lead people to live in disadvantaged neighborhoods, which can further expose them to other ambient stressors. However, their analysis was strictly quantitative and did not allow for a more nuanced analysis of how disadvantage and stress can constitute a detailed social pattern and reinforce each other in everyday life.

It is essential for stress-related research to focus on thriving. That is, given adversity, how and why do people overcome hardships and in some cases even go on to do extraordinary and exceptional things in their lives and in the lives of others? It is critical to understand how and why people experience transformative growth in the face of disadvantage in order to foster the development of positive change and empowerment among disadvantaged populations. An analysis of biographical action schemes allowed for an examination of how trajectories of suffering related to HIV were worked at to be overcome. This study advances this area of research and contributes to a more refined approach to these questions. Stigma can be a major challenge to biographical adjustment and thriving and is discussed below.

1.5   Stigma

Because HIV poses a multitude of challenges, a biographical analysis was especially useful in examining how hardship was negotiated in the current study. Those living with HIV often experience stigmatization and discrimination that can expose thelm to additional stressors and further undermine their mental and physical health (Devine et al. 1999; Herek 1999; Liu et al. 2006). According to AVERT (2010), HIV-related discrimination can occur within the domains of the government (e.g. mandatory testing, criminal sentencing for transmission of infection, restricted immigration), the healthcare system (e.g. restricted access to medication or facilities, non-consensual HIV testing, and breaches of confidentiality), employment (e.g. social isolation, termination/refusal of employment), immigration and travel (e.g. restricted entry, stay, and residence), and social exclusion in the family and community. The issue of HIV-related discrimination is a global health concern. Indeed, in approximately sixty countries, people living with HIV are faced with institutionalized discrimination hindering their access to entry, stay, and citizenship status (AVERT 2010). Recent longitudinal research utilizing a path analysis framework has demonstrated that HIV stigma among youth orphaned by AIDS in South Africa significantly predicts anxiety and depression overtime (Boyes and Cluver 2013). Their research indicates that interventions targeting stigma have great potential for improving the mental health outcomes (Boyes and Cluver 2013; Cluver et al. 2008).

   Clearly, such widespread discriminatory practices occurring in a multitude of settings can serve as stressors, exacerbating the impact of negative life events and daily stressors in the lives of those living with HIV. Three phases of the HIV/AIDS epidemic were identified by a former director of the World Health Organization (WHO), which he termed the epidemics of: (1) HIV, (2) AIDS, (3) and of stigma, discrimination, and denial (Mann 1987). Therefore, stigma has been acknowledged as an important global health concern to be targeted by program initiatives. Furthermore, the Vienna Declaration and Program of Action (1993) clearly established the importance of the protection of human rights as a major international agenda and explicitly targeted the problem of discrimination as an international human rights issue. In my study, participants perceived stigma as a structural feature which limited their freedom, basic rights, and was felt as damaging to their health and social well-being. The problem of stigma and discrimination transcended national boundaries and was made clear in this transcontinental comparison as being related to various social positions and life conditions.

Stigma remains a persistent problem of the HIV/AIDS epidemic which still has not been resolved despite decades of research and international initiatives aimed to reduce HIV stigma (Parker et al. 2002). Stigma initiatives may not have been fully effective in eliminating stigma due to the multifaceted nature of stigma rooted in social, cultural, and historical context and due to the complex, process-based nature of stigma. Below, a discussion of definitions of stigma, types of stigma, and its potential causes and consequences is provided.

The concept of stigma was introduced by Erving Goffman in his seminal work "Stigma: Notes on the Management of Spoiled Identity" as an "attribute that is deeply discrediting" which diminishes the possessor of the attribute to a discounted, tainted, and no longer whole and usual person (Goffman 1963, p. 3). Goffman (1963) emphasized the importance of the management of stigma as the management of social information present in the form of symbols, which are associated with negatively valued characteristics. Such symbols or marks were argued as varying in regards to their visibility and concealability and their degree of intrusiveness and disruption in social relationships and interaction (Goffman 1963). Goffman (1963) highlighted the role of information control in the management of stigma and strategies of concealment which can produce strain in the continual maintenance of secrecy, rendering one as not yet discredited but as having potential for discredibility. Once identified by others, the negotiation of stigma was described as a fundamental management of tension by Goffman (1963). Goffman (1963) also emphasized the importance of biography and life history as components of uniqueness forming social identity. Therefore, I focused on the biographies of PLWHA to examine how experiences rooted in biography were related to the experience of HIV stigma and the consequences of HIV stigma for identity and biographical adjustment. The strain in the maintenance of HIV as a secret draws attention to the challenges of coping with the potential for discredibility. This strain can manifest in awkwardness in interaction, a symbol of the disruptive nature of stigma in social relations (Goffman 1963; Smart and Wegner 1999).

Furthermore, Goffman (1963) distinguished three types of stigma: bodily stigma, blemishes of character, and tribal stigma. HIV is a medical condition in the body which can be marked by bodily symbols such as weight loss and which is located within the body as a virus and, therefore, constitutes a bodily stigma. HIV is an entity of its own existence that simultaneously becomes deeply embedded in the body. Also, antiretroviral therapy can contribute to conditions such as lipodystrophy which alter the body's appearance by producing extreme weight loss (lipoatrophy) or weight gain (hyperadiposity) (Collins et al. 2000; Schwenk et al. 2000). Prior research indicates that experiencing lipodystrophy and other side effects of HIV medication can affect people's self-esteem, sense of control, social and sexual relations, and can contribute to demoralization, forced disclosure, and the decision to stop treatment (Collins et al. 2000; Kremer et al. 2009). The bodily stigma and visibility of HIV can therefore be stressful and disruptive to social interaction and self-image.

Due to sexual behavior and intravenous drug use as modes of transmission for HIV, HIV is also a stigma of character that is deeply related to conceptions of morality and sin (Sandstrom 1996; UNAIDS 2005). The character-based stigma associating HIV with sin and sexuality can correspond to attributions of blame for the cause of HIV infection and to social rejection, judgment, and distance from people with HIV (Parker et al. 2002; UNAIDS 2005). Prior research suggests that PLWHA are blamed for their HIV infection and that they are more severely blamed when their infection is due to sexual behavior or injection drug use (Herek and Capitanio 1999). Previous studies also indicate that PLWHA experience more stigma than people living with cancer, which suggests that the dimensions of blame and beliefs about the cause of illness play important roles in stigma (Idemudia and Matamela 2012; Greene and Banerjee 2006).

Attributions of blame can intensify stigma towards PLWHA. HIV can be conceived of as a tribal stigma, linking a person to membership in a socially deviant group of people with HIV and also of at-risk groups for HIV such as the gay community, racial/ethnic minorities, and other marginalized social groups. Gay men are blamed more for their HIV infection than their heterosexual counterparts and African Americans are blamed more for their HIV than their white counterparts regardless of gender (Herek and Capitanio 1999).

These attributions of blame and stereotypes can reinforce preexisting social inequality because marginalized groups are symbolically linked to conceptions of HIV, perpetuating negative attitudes and justifications for social exclusion. For example, Link and Phelan (2006) emphasized the role of power in their conceptualization of stigma as a process involving components of (1) identifying and labeling differences, (2) stereotyping where one is linked to undesirable characteristics, (3) the group labeling makes a distinction between "us" versus "them," (4) those stigmatized experience discrimination and status loss, and (5) the exercise of power. Link and Phelan's (2006) conceptualization of stigma emphasizes the role of power and social, economic, and cultural resources in stigma. Those who are stigmatized lack the power to challenge their marginalization and those who enforce stigma can possess the power to maintain socially unequal relationships. Accordingly, there can be a layering of stigma, where multiple stigmas intersect (Parker et al. 2002).

The integral role of the body in the management of stigma indicates that for PLWHA, their bodies can become a place of social controversy. The body can become a politicized space seen as needing containment and control by medical institutions and as a vehicle or weapon for the transmission of the virus. The moral and political discourses surrounding HIV can also serve to de-sexualize PLWHA's bodies and identities by making PLWHA feel that their sexual lives are fundamentally changed and existentially threatened (Sandstrom 1996; Siegel and Krauss 1991). Prior research suggests that visual imagery associated with the embodiment of HIV such as images of: death, sex, sin, fragmentation, isolation, dangerousness, out of one's control, and in need of containment can contribute to HIV stigma (Varas-Díaz and Toro-Alfonso 2003). Rejection has been conceptualized as a form of betrayal (Strauss 1997). Experiences of rejection can serve to exacerbate feelings of sexual undesirability and even the potential death of a highly valued aspect of the self, one's sexual identity.

Another major focus of this analysis was how the concept of stigma was experienced by participants and how their experiences could elaborate the concept of stigma. Sub-themes of stigma that emerged in these narratives, such as stigma that was anticipated, experienced, proliferated to intimate others, and the roles of appearance in shaping interaction were emphasized. These dimensions of stigma were similar to those of felt, enacted, and secondary stigma discussed here. The role of visibility and appearance in stigma was emphasized in narrators' experiences. The role of body weight as a symbolic marker of HIV status and its importance in shaping interaction emerged as an important element of participants' experiences of stigma. The body is a fundamental condition shaping social interaction that often is taken for granted. However, appearance was an emergent theme in the narratives which emerged without any solicitation.

The emphasis placed on body weight or "thinness" as a marker of HIV and of the importance of attractiveness in allowing people to "pass" as being HIV-negative highlights the importance of the body as an object to self and others as posited by Anselm Strauss (Strauss 1993). Because HIV status can be hidden in the absence of noticeable changes in appearance, when such alterations in appearance were experienced they were discussed as a mark of HIV status and illness and as provoking negative treatment by others and a great deal of emotional distress.

Strauss (1993) made explicit the role of the body in social interaction when he argued that when the self is involved with the body, we begin to relate to our own bodies as objects and others also react to our bodies. The body can thus be seen as a condition for social interaction and as having its own set of processes, which play a role in how the body shapes interaction and problematic social interaction. For Strauss, mental activity and the body are intertwined and there are contextual conditions for the body in interaction, which include the body state and biographical moment of action (Strauss 1993). Body weight and attractiveness may thus be defined as contextual conditions for social interaction that appear to be especially critical in biographical moments of crisis. Appearance emerged as essential to social interaction as it related to HIV stigma in this study. The roles of the body and the symbolic meaning ascribed to bodily states as they relate to self-image, other's reactions towards people with HIV, and representation of self are further discussed in the comparison chapters.

Stigma may constitute a "self-fulfilling prophecy" defined by Robert Merton as "a false definition of the situation evoking a new behavior which makes the originally false conception come true" (Merton 1968, p. 477). Symbolic interaction theorists have emphasized the importance of other's perceptions and actions in shaping identity and behavior. For example, George H. Mead (Mead 1934) focused on the creation of social order through social interaction and how social actors, through their interpretations of social situations and communication with others, give meaning to social interaction. Also, Charles H. Cooley's (Cooley 1902) discussion of the "looking glass self" emphasizes the importance of an individual's perception of how others perceive them in shaping their self-perception. Accordingly, social exchange theory, which emphasizes social interaction as a mutually reinforcing process over time where structures involve long-term relations between people and power is unequally distributed, can be applied to the study of stigma because stigma can be negotiated by actors in social interaction over time (Emerson 1976; Gramling and Forsyth 1987). Contemporary sociologists have continued to emphasize the importance of social meaning and internalization of other's perceptions in defining the self. For example, according to Link and colleagues (Link et al. 1989) in their modified labeling theory, prior to entry in a stigmatized status, people are aware of negative stereotypes and public conceptions of the given position and have internalized these conceptions.

Consistent with a symbolic interactionist approach and modified labeling theory, prior studies suggest that stigma can be internalized (Crocker and Major 1989; Parker et al. 2002). Felt or perceived stigma can occur even in the absence of overt discrimination (Jacoby 1994). Felt stigma can contribute to a host of adverse affective responses such as shame, embarrassment, and self-blame (UNAIDS 2005). Felt stigma can also motivate people to avoid stigma by isolating themselves and avoiding social interaction when they paradoxically need support from others (UNAIDS 2005). Therefore, felt stigma is an important component of stigma that should be understood from people's experiences and their constructions of meaning. Felt stigma can serve as a barrier to biographical adjustment to HIV by producing fear and avoidance among PLWHA. Accordingly, prior research suggests that fear of stigma can be a barrier to engagement in treatment and prevention (Kalichman and Simbayi 2003; Lichtenstein et al. 2005; Mahajan et al. 2008). Enacted stigma corresponds to the phase of stigma involving discrimination identified by Link and Phelan (2006). The experience of discrimination or enacted stigma can serve to reaffirm feelings of stigma and to damage people's self-concepts and relationships. The distinction between felt and enacted stigma is useful because it draws attention to the possibility that stigma does not always result in discrimination because discrimination can depend on power dynamics (Link and Phelan 2006).

In addition, German sociologist Gerhard Falk (Falk 2001) identified two types of outsiders: the "existential" and the "achieved." Existential outsiders were defined as those who are stigmatized due to the essential nature of their existence, regardless of their actions. Falk defined achieved outsiders as those whose actions or life conditions result in stigma. Based on Falk's (2001) definition of existential and achieved stigma, HIV can be conceived of as both existential due to the existential threat to mortality and morality HIV poses and as achieved due to sexual behavior and injection drug use as potential modes of transmission. HIV diagnosis can be especially stressful in the context of stigma and negative stereotypes that people must integrate into their pre-existing conceptions of HIV and of themselves. Chronic illness can lead to biographical disruption and undermine former conceptions of self and life plans (Charmaz 1983; 1995; McCann et al. 2010). HIV can present an existential threat upon diagnosis due to an initial fear of death and to threat to self, social relationships, and social status

(Charmaz 1983; Siegel and Krauss 1991). A biographical analysis of how HIV is integrated into biography and the biographical work involved in adaptation to living with HIV can help expand understanding of how people live with and negotiate stigma.

Jones et al. (1984), drawing on Goffman's (1963) discussion of the link between attributes and stereotypes, argued that stigma constitutes a mark linking its possessor to undesirable characteristics and stereotypes. According to Jones et al. (1984), stigma involves six components: (1) concealability, (2) course of the mark, (3) disruptiveness, (4) aesthetics, (5) origin, and (6) peril. These components of stigma parallel and extend Goffman's (1963) conceptualization of stigma. The importance of concealability corresponds to Goffman's (1963) discussion of visibility and the emphasis on aesthetics further argues for the importance of physical appearance and the body in stigma. Research indicates that concealment of stigma in interaction can be stressful, intruding into one's thoughts and contributing to feelings of secrecy (Smart and Wegner 1999). In addition, the dimension of origin in stigma emphasizes the importance about the etiology of stigmatized conditions. For example, causal attributions of the etiology of mental illness have been found to be related to preferences to social distance and social control of mental illness in recent research (Mossakowski et al. 2011). The dimension of peril or of threat and dangerousness has also been linked to stigma in mental illness research (Link et al. 1999; Pescosolido et al. 1999). The origin of a stigma can invoke attributions of blame by assigning responsibility (Gramling and Forsyth 1987).

Anti-stigma initiatives have targeted fear of infection by providing education about the route of HIV transmission and have reduced stigma but have not eliminated it (Brown et al. 2003). Potentially, providing medical information about HIV may serve only to reduce the stigma of the body and not address the stigma of character attached to HIV. Prior research indicates that attributing the cause of other deviant statuses such as mental illness to biological causes does not reduce stigma and actually predicts preferences for social distance and social control (Mossakowski et al. 2011). Therefore, understanding how stigma intersects with different social positions and statuses rooted in socio-historical context and personal biography can help to develop a multidimensional conceptualization of stigma. Due to the multidimensional nature of stigma, anti-stigma interventions which target only fear of infection may not be comprehensive.

Others have distinguished between tangible and symbolic threat (Stangor and Crandall 2000). Tangible threat involves fear of death or infection whereas symbolic threat threatens moral sentiments. The moral dimensions ascribed to suffering can affect how people are treated (Charmaz 1999). HIV presents both a tangible threat as an infectious disease and symbolic threat disrupting moral sentiments. Tangible and symbolic threats are embedded in medical and public discourse, respectively. The symbolic threat of HIV as representing sexual and moral irresponsibility and sinful action can be perpetuated in religious settings and cannot be addressed unless there are challenges to such discourse. However, due to the shame and secrecy of HIV, such challenges to discourse can be hindered thus preventing social change in conceptions of HIV. The moral and affective components of HIV stigma must be placed into social context in order to address stigma by others and to understand how PLWHA navigate the fearful and rejecting actions of those motivated by instrumental and symbolic threats. Variations in stigma may be rooted in social, historical, and cultural context, thus encouraging cross-cultural studies of HIV stigma. Stigma can even proliferate to intimate others or to those working the HIV/AIDS field thus constituting what Goffman (1963) termed a "courtesy stigma" which has also been described as a secondary stigma (Cao et al. 2006; Ogunmefun et al. 2011).

Stigma and experiences of discrimination are inherently stressful, with prior research demonstrating linkages between stigma and negative mental health outcomes and as limiting life chances in terms of employment and integration into the community (Link et al. 2008; Link and Phelan, 2001; Lai et al. 2001; Markowitz, 1998). Such discriminatory practices can arise from fear and a lack of understanding about conditions such as mental illness and HIV (Corrigan et al. 2003; Herek 1999; Markowitz 1998; Pescosolido et al. 1999). While negative attitudes regarding HIV have been examined, the intricacies in biographical processes and social interactions involved in HIV-related stigma and discrimination remain an important issue for researchers (Parker and Aggleton 2003). How are stigma and discrimination experienced? How is stigma related to social networks and support? What are its antecedents and consequences? How are stigma and discrimination effectively negotiated? Understanding the context of stigma and discrimination as well as understanding how they are coped with can help shed light on these questions. HIV stigma is not experienced in a social vacuum, people with HIV can possess other social statuses that can exacerbate or mitigate the stress of experiencing HIV stigma. By applying a biographical analysis, HIV stigma can be examined as it is rooted in personal and cultural context.

In addition to discriminatory practices and social exclusion, many of those living with HIV face socioeconomic disadvantage, which can further undermine their well-being and limit their life chances (Greene et al. 2006). Prior research shows that socioeconomic disadvantage is associated with impaired mental and physical health (McLeod and Shanahan 1996; Miech et al. 1999). According to social stress theory, disadvantage can differentially expose those in lower social positions to stressors and heighten their vulnerability to such stressors (Pearlin 1989).

Specifically, social positions rooted in structural arrangements can play a key role in differential exposure to stressors and access to mediators (e.g. coping resources and social support), affecting vulnerability to stress (Aneshensel 1992; Pearlin 1989; Turner et al. 1995). Interestingly, while social stress theory has been applied to various stressors, this framework has not been extensively applied in the field of HIV-related research. Research utilizing a biographical approach can address this gap in the literature. Stressors do not exist in isolation, and for PLWHA, the constellation of multiple stressors is especially relevant. This is because not only of its relevance in health-related research, but also because it provides an opportunity to focus on how experiences at multiple levels of social reality can interact with one another, potentially damaging well-being and quality of life.

Also, perceived stress has been shown to be associated with a range of negative outcomes, such as impaired mental health, negative health-related behaviors, and self-reported health (Bovier et al. 2004). There is a substantial body of research in regards to HIV and coping in the psychological literature (Antoni et al. 1991; Billings et al. 2000; Ironson et al. 1994; Ironson et al. 2005; Leserman et al. 2000; Mulder et al. 1995; Solano et al. 2002). Indeed, research shows that social support is positively associated with adherence to medication (Kremer et al. 2006) and that avoidant coping is associated with disease progression among people living with HIV (Antoni et al. 1991; Billings et al. 2000; Ironson et al. 1994; Ironson et al. 2005; Leserman et al. 2000; Mulder et al. 1995; Solano et al. 2002). Therefore, additional research is needed which applies a social stress framework to the study of coping with HIV. Furthermore, the social causation hypothesis suggests that social stressors rooted in disadvantaged social positions can lead to impaired functioning (Dohrenwend and Dohrenwend 1969; Dohrenwend et al. 1992). Examining how the stigmatized social status of HIV intersects with other social statuses such as socioeconomic status, race/ethnicity, and sexual orientation can help to develop an understanding of how social processes of marginalization can "get under the skin" and disrupt lives. Chronic, ongoing stress rooted in socially unequal positions can wear down the body's stress response over time, resulting in allostatic load which further erodes the body's ability to manage stress (McEwen 2002). Accordingly, race/ ethnicity and immigration status can be related to the experience of stress which can be pronounced among PLWHA.

1.6   Race/Ethnicity and Migration Context

Prior research suggests that ethnicity is related to views of HIV and medicine. For example, in a study of men and woman living with HIV in Texas, USA, researchers found that African Americans and Latinos were more likely to believe in HIV as a genocidal conspiracy, and believing in HIV as a genocidal conspiracy was associated with having sex without using condoms (Ross et al. 2006). Race/ ethnicity and socioeconomic status also have been found to have interactive effects on psychological distress and health in the United States, which emphasizes the intersectionality of these social positions (Kessler and Neighbors 1986; Williams and Collins 1995) Research also indicates that African American men are subject to more stigma than their White and Latino counterparts among Gay communities (Smit et al. 2011). Because the United States has a unique history rooted in slavery, racial segregation, and racial conflict, comparing the experiences between people in the United States and Germany can help to clarify how historical racism shapes illness experience and treatment (Bayor 2003; Massey and Denton 1993).

Germany also has a history characterized by racism, and then, during the Nazi regime, genocide. Substantial immigration from other nations over the last decades makes both nations useful in generating comparative insights (Hansen 2003; Boswell 2003). Due to the international nature of the recruitment setting in Germany, my sample included migrants from different African nations, Turkey, and native Germans. The sample in the United States included African Americans, Latinos, and Whites. This allowed for a comparison of the experiences of people from different countries of origin, different host countries and contexts of immigration.

In Europe, Germany has been identified as one of the countries that has one of the highest proportions of people with HIV from endemic countries, with ethnic minorities being an at-risk group (Del Amo et al. 2001). Germany is a nation characterized by large spatial boundaries, a large population of approximately 81 million, a powerful economy, and substantial immigration (Hansen 2003; OECDa 2012; Siebert 2003). The German economy is the fourth largest in the world, has a major influence on other nation's economies, and has rebounded despite recent economic challenges (OECDa, 2012). The topic of immigration and economic security and growth is an ongoing political debate with public surveys suggesting that the German public has a concern of the impact of immigration on social security resources and holds negative attitudes towards migrants (The Local, 2012; Abali, 2009). These fears and negative attitudes towards immigration can minimize the potential positive impact immigration could have on Germany. For instance, due to a decrease in population growth in Germany immigration may have the potential to contribute to the nation's economic growth by meeting population deficits in employment sectors (OECD 2012a).

Approximately, 25 percent of migrants in Germany immigrate from the European Union nations with a substantial number coming from Italy and Greece, over 25 percent come from other European nations such as the former Yugoslavia and Poland (Haug et al. 2002; Seibert 2003). Another quarter come from Turkey and the rest come from Asia (12 percent), Africa (4 percent) and the Americas (3 percent) (Haug et al. 2002; Siebert 2003). Germany has an enduring history of immigration with substantial immigration from other nations and more recent movement within the nation occurring post World War II after the reunification of West and East Germany in 1989 (Hansen 2003). Immigrants tend to migrate to West Germany and major metropolitan areas, with 10.4 percent of the population in West Germany being foreign born, which is equivalent to the foreign born population in the United States (Siebert 2003). West Germany has a substantial migrant population (Haug et al. 2002; Wienold et al. 2007). West Germany and Berlin have substantial migrant populations with 96 percent of all migrants residing in West Germany and Berlin; 41 percent of all migrants have been estimated to reside in Frankfurt (IOM 2007; Wienold et al. 2007). Approximately 430,000 asylum seekers reside in West Germany and receive benefits. Over 5 million asylum seekers, mostly coming from other European nations, Asia, and Africa, sought refuge in Western Europe between 1985 and 1999 and almost half of these asylum seekers came to Germany (Haug et al. 2002). As discussed in the results section, policies regarding asylum seeking and immigration can have a major impact on the experience of living with HIV by shaping the spatial and local context of patient's lives because displacement programs geared at reducing the costs of asylum seekers involve involuntary placement in certain locations of Germany (Boswell 2003).

The common and yet contested nature of immigration in Germany make it impossible to ignore the importance of immigration context as it relates to the experience of living with HIV. The challenges faced by migrants, particularly asylum seekers, of facing poverty, living in overcrowded housing, and of discrimination have been documented by the United Nations as a social and human rights concern (UN 2012). Migrants have been recognized as an underserved population in Germany's HIV/AIDS prevention and treatment initiatives (Wienold et al. 2007; IOM 2007). In 2006, migrants from countries with high HIV/AIDS prevalence became the second largest at-risk group for HIV in Germany and continue to be an at-risk group for HIV infection (Wienold et al. 2007; UNAIDS 2012). According to UNAIDS (2012), migrants coming from countries with high HIV prevalence, men who have sex with men (MSM), and injection drug users (IDUs) are the largest at-risk groups for HIV in Germany. MSMs represent a majority of HIV infections in Germany (Bätzing-Feigenbaum et al. 2008; Wienold et al. 2007; UNAIDS 2012). However, the incidence of HIV infection is increasing among women and decreasing for men (Wienold et al. 2007). Women who have migrated to Germany from high prevalence countries are disproportionately diagnosed with HIV relative to their percentage of the population (Wienold et al. 2007). Heterosexual contact is the predominant mode of transmission for women in Germany and in other nations (European Centre for Disease Prevention and Control 2011). Women with HIV require special medical attention in part due to their need for prenatal and maternal medical care; the German health care system appears to be effective in providing such care because HIV due to mother-to-child transmission of HIV in Germany is estimated to be less than 1 percent (UNAIDS 2012). Prevalence of HIV among IDUs has decreased and may be a positive outcome of needle exchange programs geared at the prevention of HIV transmission and other blood-borne pathogens (UNAIDS 2012). The coordination of public and private services and the mainstreaming or integration of HIV as a concern for programs in different sectors such as education, the workplace, and medical care in Germany appears to be helpful in effectively addressing the HIV/AIDS epidemic, but the issue of HIV among migrants remains a major challenge (GIZ 2012; UNAIDS 2012; IOM 2007). The overall prevalence of HIV in Germany has increased due to decreased mortality and increased rate of new HIV infections which suggests that care needs to be targeted towards those living with HIV for long periods of time and towards prevention of new infections (UNAIDS 2012).

My sample included both newly diagnosed patients and those living for decades with HIV. No participants in my sample recruited in Germany were reported injection drug users. However, the absence of a more detailed discussion of past and current drug use could be due to social desirability bias with interviewees minimizing any past or current IDU-status. While not applicable to all participants, past drug use was alluded to by some participants who described living prior lifestyles characterized by high-risk behavior or "sex, drugs, and rock and roll." Another possibility is that current IDUs were not participating in treatment at the clinic and were either seeking help elsewhere or were not seeking treatment. Frankfurt is characterized by a unique context where IDUs have access to drug consumption rooms where they can consume drugs in a private and safe setting where personnel and other drug users are provided training to help them detect symptoms of overdose and to understand the importance of using sterile injection materials (Deutsche AIDS-Hilfe e.V 2011). The provision of legal protection and drug use services could also direct IDUs to medical treatment, making it more likely for IDUs to receive specialist care. AIDS-Hilfe Frankfurt e.V. (a non-partisan organization) was created in reaction to the stigma surrounding the emergence of AIDS cases in Germany in the mid 1980s and currently is in operation. AIDS-Hilfe e.V. provides a variety of resources and services for PLWHA such as HIV testing, referrals to treatment, and information regarding drug consumption rooms, legal advice, and medical consultations for drug users. Despite this context of a more progressive and tolerant drug policy in Frankfurt, while some participants alluded to a history of drug use, no one interviewed in Frankfurt explicitly discussed being an IDU. Perhaps despite these initiatives for IDUS and PLWHA, interviewees still felt drug use to be discrediting and may have therefore focused more on their HIV than drug use. Another possibility is because the narrative interviews were focused on living with HIV, interviewees may have focused more on HIV because they felt this was more important in the context of the interviews. The importance of the structure of interviews and its relationship to findings is discussed in more detail in the methodology and discussion chapters.

In addition to Frankfurt's progressive drug policy, there are a number of characteristics that make Frankfurt a valuable research location. Metropolitan areas have higher HIV prevalence than less densely populated areas and incidence of HIV infection, and Hamburg, Berlin, and Munich have the highest rates of AIDS prevalence in Germany (Wienold et al. 2007). Also, research suggests that Hamburg, Berlin, Stuttgart, Munich, and Frankfurt had high rates of newly diagnosed cases of HIV which highlights the importance of interviewing patients in an urban setting (Bätzing-Feigenbaum et al. 2008). Importantly, a substantial percentage of HIV infections among migrants have been estimated to occur in Germany and not abroad (Wienold et al. 2007). Among men who have sex with men (MSM), approximately 51 percent are estimated to be of German origin and nationality (Wienold et al. 2007). Notably, there is no law in Germany forbidding the entry and stay of people with

HIV/AIDS (IOM 2007). The demographic characteristics of my sample recruited in Germany correspond to these estimates including MSM who were white men of German origin and women both native to Germany and who had immigrated from African nations and Turkey. Article 3 of the German Constitution ensures the right of non-discrimination. Public opinion surveys suggest that stigma against PLWHA may have decreased in Germany but this stigma in public attitudes continues to be a major social problem (UNAIDS 2012).

Similar to Germany, the United States is characterized by its large spatial boundaries and sizable population of over 300 million, and enduring immigration (U.S. Census Bureau 2013). Although the USA and Germany are similar with both being large and powerful nations characterized by immigration, there are unique migration contexts in both nations, with each nation having different immigration policies and immigration from different countries. Importantly, there is substantial inequality in insurance coverage for foreign-born versus US citizens (Department of Homeland Security 2009). In the USA, immigration has shifted from being primarily European to being characterized by migration from Asia, Latin countries, and the Caribbean. In 2011, the majority of legal permanent residents were those born in Mexico, China, and India (Department of Homeland Security 2012a). Asylum seekers also constitute a substantial number of migrants: 56,384 people were admitted to the USA as refugees and 24,988 were granted asylum in 2011 (Department of Homeland Security 2012b). Approximately 75 percent of refugees came from Burma, Bhutan, and Iraq and many others came from Somalia, Cuba, Eritrea, Iran, and the Democratic Republic of Congo (Department of Homeland Security 2012b). Those granted asylum came mostly from China, Venezuela, and Ethiopia and those from China, Nepal, and Haiti also received a large number of travel documents while abroad allowing their entry to the USA (Department of Homeland Security 2012b). States with the largest refugee resident populations include Florida, New York, Texas, and California (Department of Homeland Security 2012b). Miami is one of the leading metropolitan areas in the USA with a large population of immigrants (Department of Homeland Security 2009b).

After World War II, the cities of Los Angeles, Miami, San Diego, and Houston became major gateways for migration (The Brookings Institution 2004). By 2000, Miami experienced the sharpest growth in its foreign-born population among these gateway cities with a large movement of Cuban refugees into Miami, with foreign-born residents reaching 60 percent of the population in 2000 and immigration driving Miami's population growth (The Brookings Institution 2004). Miami is racially and ethnically diverse, with a large African American

and Hispanic population (US Census Bureau 2013). Unfortunately, Miami is also
characterized by high levels of income inequality and residential segregation
(Pew 2012). Residential segregation can perpetuate poverty and racism,
reinforcing social inequality (Massey and Denton 1993).

Socioeconomic disadvantage is a major issue for PLWHA in the U.S., with
rates of HIV prevalence being higher among those living in poverty and
disadvantaged groups having disproportionate rates of HIV infection (Denning
2010). The relationship between poverty and HIV emphasizes the importance of
cost-reduction for HIV treatment for patients. Insurance coverage for HIV
medication can also be problematic due to the high cost of medication and
limited coverage. Insurance coverage can affect continuity of care. For example,
prior research suggests that eligibility for antiretroviral treatment is related to
continuity of care among HIV patients (Torian and Wiewel 2011). Organizations
such as the Ryan White Foundation and social security can help to cover the cost
of HIV treatment but the requirements to meet coverage for AIDS Drug
Assistance Programs (ADAPs) often include a low-income and filing for
disability or discontinuing full-time employment. Barack Obama's recent reform
of heath care policy under the Affordable Care Act (ACA) may help PLWHA by
removing the disability requirement to qualify for Medicaid coverage, which is
the largest source of HIV medical coverage in the United States (Kaiser Family
Foundation 2012). The ACA also makes it illegal for health insurance companies
to deny coverage based on pre-existing conditions including HIV. Also, the ACA
amends current health care policies so that ADAPs can be covered under
Medicare, reducing the cost of HIV medication for patients. The recent national
attention to the issue of health care and to the importance of developing a
national strategy for HIV/AIDS highlights the importance of comparative
research between the USA and other countries with different health care systems.
The interview site in Miami provided a unique opportunity for a comparison of
interviews between Frankfurt and Miami.

Rates of HIV infection in Miami have been estimated to be some of the
highest the United States and over 30 percent of the population in Miami has
been estimated to lack health insurance (Florida Department of Health 2009). In
2009, Miami was ranked as number one in the country with the highest number
of new AIDS cases per capita and the neighboring Broward County, Fort
Lauderdale area ranked second in new AIDS cases in the United States (Florida
Department of Health 2009). Miami has also been noted for its "culture of
excess" where hedonism and the constant pursuit of pleasure and stimulation are
widespread, which may lend the area to a social context particularly conducive to

high risk behavior such as drug use and unsafe sexual practices (Gaines 2009). The state of Florida ranked third in the nation in the number of people living with AIDS and second for the number of pediatric AIDS cases (Florida Department of Health 2009). Similar to Germany, the majority of HIV/AIDS cases in the USA are among men but are increasing among women, and in Miami MSMs constitute a majority of HIV-cases (Florida Department of Health 2009).

Rates of HIV are disproportionately higher among African Americans and Hispanics than for their non-Hispanic white counterparts, and AIDS is a major leading cause of death for African Americans and Hispanics, and pediatric cases of HIV/AIDS involve a majority of African Africans in Florida (Florida Department of Health 2009). National estimates indicate that African Americans accounted for 46 percent of HIV infections in 2010 (CDC 2012). In 2009, the highest rate of death due to AIDS was that for blacks/African Americans with a rate of 29.3 per 100,000 population (CDC 2012). Between 2007 and 2009, the rates of death due to AIDS in the U.S. increased among Asians, whites, and those reporting multiple races (CDC 2012). Clearly, HIV is a major health problem in the U.S. and in the Miami, Florida region, which disproportionately affects racial/ ethnic minorities. With high income inequality and residential segregation, racial/ ethnic and cultural diversity, and inequality in insurance coverage between migrants and natives, HIV is a major problem in Miami, making Miami an ideal location to examine how PLWHA negotiate their health.

Importantly, prior to 2010, HIV was listed on the Center for Disease Control's (CDC) list of communicable diseases of public significance which required mandatory testing and prohibited entry and stay, thus preventing PLWHA from obtaining a legal permanent residence (LPR) status or green card and citizenship (Brown and Cetron 2011). The recent changes to lift the immigration ban on HIV have received considerable attention in the media and in public discourse. Therefore, a comparison to nations such as Germany that do not have laws prohibiting immigration due to HIV status can help to generate insights into migration experience and how it immigration policy can affect living with HIV. Fear of detection of HIV status can be a major barrier to HIV treatment which can be pronounced due to fears of deportation. In contrast, an immigration policy that encourages testing and treatment without fear of deportation can play a critical role in migrant's medical treatment.

Despite being a wealthy, industrialized nation, the United States is characterized by high income inequality, relative poverty, and a health care system that has recently undergone social reform (OECD 2012b; Kaiser Family Foundation 2012).

Comparative research is needed because the conditions and experiences of patients may vary considerably cross-culturally affecting suffering and illness trajectories. As a dimension of social conditions, health policies are highly consequential for persons living with HIV. Also, in light of the recent 2008 recession and the continued difficulties in the United States to stabilize the economy, it is crucial to understand how health care experiences can inform policy (OECD 2012b). Experiences of illness can be examined using the biographical approach which focuses on deep, internal processes in relation to personal and collective history. The U.S. has a unique history involving the genocide of Native Americans, the slavery of African Americans, immigration, and enduring social inequality and racial conflict. These persistent inequalities are rendered even more visible in the case of HIV which disproportionately affects minorities and those living in poverty. In addition, the health care system, with its disability and low-income requirements for HIV treatment could continue to perpetuate health and social inequality. Using biographical analysis, this study examines how such a history is embedded in personal experience with HIV.

Both nations have histories of racism, but these histories are distinct in their specific events and characteristics and occurred in unique cultural contexts which have shaped both nations' more recent histories and the relations within their boundaries. The importance of history in understanding the sociocultural context of patients' experiences is pronounced through the use of a comparative study. Accordingly, important elements of a nation's sociocultural context are its approach to social policy and to the treatment of various racial/ethnic groups. The German health care system is distinct from that of the United States, allowing for a contrast and comparison of sociocultural context and policy.

A nation's social policies can be conceptualized as representative of its socio-cultural and ideological approaches. While both the nations can be considered individualistic, Germany's sense of social responsibility and emphasis on the importance of social security appears to manifest in its comprehensive medical insurance, unemployment, and pension provision although the debate surrounding the provision of social security is becoming a rising concern. In contrast, the U.S. minimizes the need and responsibility of the government to provide such social security in a social context where there is a strong belief in a meritocratic and equal opportunity structure, which justifies denying fundamental rights such as health care coverage by blaming those who do not succeed economically and socially for their limitations. Furthermore, in the American health care system, health is treated as a market place commodity, and this allows for the dominance of private insurance and pharmaceutical companies in health care. In the U.S., Medicaid coverage extends to only about half of people with HIV for medical care and in order to qualify for coverage people were required to be on disability until the ACA policy change (Kaiser Family Foundation 2012).

The recent changes to U.S. health care effective in 2014 will remove the disability requirement for eligibility but require an income of $14,000 or less. This requirement to be in poverty can be problematic for PLWHA who need HIV insurance coverage but who are employed and would like to earn wages that provide them with a quality of life above poverty-level and could also be a disincentive for those in poverty to work to increase their incomes and rise out of poverty due to concerns of losing their medical coverage. For private insurance coverage, these reforms are expected to increase the availability and reduce the cost of private insurance for those earning $15,000-45,000 a year.

In Germany, recent policy developments such as the implementation of the Hartz reforms, which limited social welfare benefits, have been a source of heated debate within Germany as critics argue that the Hartz reforms are an infringement on basic human rights guaranteed by the German government (The Guardian 2013). Also, in the context of rising income inequality and of high levels of unemployment and poverty in Germany the importance of examining social welfare policies including health care coverage is made especially clear for both policy makers and patients (UN 2012; OECD 2012c).

These political debates also emphasize transnational research as a priority in the context of social policy changes in the U.S. The U.S. health care reform makes strides against prior discrimination by insurance companies making it illegal to deny coverage or to charge higher rates for people with pre-existing conditions, including HIV, and by making changes to cut the cost of HIV medication premiums for those with Medicare. The ACA is also planned to implement community-based changes by providing care for those uninsured by increasing community health centers and their medical staff. However, at the time of this study these changes had not yet taken effect. Regardless, as the U.S. is on the verge of implementing a vast health care reform, the experiences of PLWHA are nonetheless important in order to further inform potential avenues for improving health care policy with a patient-focused approach on their experiences with HIV. Many of the people interviewed in Miami were living in poverty and forced to go on disability in order to qualify for their medical coverage. In contrast to Frankfurt, economic hardship and perpetual poverty rooted in social inequalities were problems which interviewees in Miami had to overcome and which were related to their medical care. A comparison of cases in the two locations helped to generate insights and to highlight social context in biographical experience as it was rooted in personal and collective history and life conditions.

The use of in-depth qualitative analysis of biographical data can help to demonstrate how meaning is actively constructed in social relations. The biographical approach allows for an examination of how social meaning is given to a subject's everyday life (Bertaux and Kohli 1984; Chanfrault-Duchet 1995). This approach is well suited for the goals of this study because it enables a focus on life trajectories rooted in their social contexts, allowing for the discovery of social processes which can influence patterns of social relations (Bertaux and Kohli 1984). A comparison of the two distinct samples in different locations allowed for new insights to be generated that were rooted in local context.

In order to discuss the roles of stigma and coping in relation to stress, health, and broader societal conditions, I applied a biographical analysis guided by the theoretical and methodological approaches of Anselm Strauss and of Fritz Schütze. This approach allowed me to identify biographical processes related to coping, identity, and stigma. My analysis began with a discussion of participant's descriptions of their biographies as they unfolded. In my analysis, the initial HIV diagnosis was examined and participant's emotions and reactions to their HIV diagnosis were discussed. While using a constant comparative approach, I utilized the analytical concepts of the trajectory of suffering (Riemann and Schütze 1991) and biographical process structures of action and transformation to analyze participants' narratives. That is, how did participants become aware of their own agency and by what processes were they motivated to utilize their agency to improve their life conditions? Below is a discussion of the methodology used in this study and the process of comparison.

2 Biographical Analysis Using Narrative and Topical Interviews

2.1 Brief History of Biographical Methodology, Debates, and Developments

The use of biographical methodology grew in the 1960s as researchers became increasingly concerned with the importance of personal and social meanings as a basis for action and critiqued positivist approaches as being detached from lived reality (Chamberlayne et al. 2000). Researchers focused on the debates of the relationship between agency and social structure and felt that despite Gidden's (1995) contribution of structuration theory to help clarify the link between agency and social structure, their linkage remained insufficiently clarified. The search to identify research methods that examined multiple aspects of social reality drove a "turn" to biographical methodology (Chamberlayne et al. 2000). Biographical research provides a means of relating micro- and macro- levels of social reality which are rooted in personal and collective history.

Both historians and sociologists began to recognize personal narratives as a viable means to understanding society and social change. This development to biographical research brought to attention the need to develop an understanding of the relations between agency and meaning and the role of memory and identity. In the early 1980s debates about memory questioned empiricism and the ability of biographical research to generate meaningful insights (Chamberlayne et al. 2000). These debates brought up questions about the nature and role of subjectivity in biographical methodology and allowed for a response to these criticisms and to the further development of biographical methods. Some of the criticisms launched at biographical methodology were driven by postmodernist assertions that individual accounts were not real, that subjective accounts were arbitrary, and that all that such accounts could provide were an analysis of text in the present moment in time. Biographical research was even criticized as being ahistorical, which presented a major challenge to biographical research. However, these criticisms have since then been addressed. For example, in the 1990s, biographical researchers increasingly emphasized the importance of history in understanding human beings and their actions. As Chamberlayne et al. (2000) explained:

> "To understand oneself and others, we need to understand our own histories and how we have become who we are. We make our own history but not under conditions of our own choosing, and we need to understand these conditions of action more if our future making of our own making is to produce outcomes closer to our intentions and projects." (p. 7)

Accordingly, as Chamberlayne et al. (2000) described, biographical researchers strive to:

> "Describe people as historically formed actors whose biographies are necessary to render fully intelligible their historical action in context – in conditions, meanings and outcomes, whether such conditions, meanings and outcomes be conscious or unconscious." (p. 8)

As a shift which strengthened the relationship between psychoanalysis and the social sciences developed, the focus on further understanding agency began to overcome the postmodernist criticisms of subjectivity (Chamberlayne et al. 2000). Instead, subjectivity was seen as a means of providing "thick description" of human beings as individuals whose actions were influenced by historical forces and so personal accounts were acknowledged as a means of accessing personal meaning rooted in historical context (Geertz 1973). In Germany, a shift from life course research to biographical analysis occurred and biographical research associations were established which further legitimized the biographical approach (Apitzsch and Inowlocki 2000). The genesis of the biographical approach developed in a context of transnational interchange between the United States, Germany, and France (Apitzsch and Inowlocki 2000). Apitzsch and Inowlocki's (2000) discussion of the development of biographical methodology (further discussed below) emphasized the deep inter-relational character of theory and method.

Debates of subjectivity and its relationship to knowledge such as the argument that truth could not be determined from subjective accounts and that researchers were over-interpreting such accounts have been raised against biographical analysis. However, in response to these criticisms, researchers such as Fritz Schütze further developed the biographical method and thus addressed these criticisms and advanced the biographical approach (Apitzsch and Inowlocki 2000). Because Fritz Schütze argued that cases should be analyzed not only sequentially but in terms of representation and meaning, and because he developed empirically based concepts which could be analyzed in a systematic manner such as biographical process structures, he helped to advance biographical research beyond these criticisms.

Process structures are related to life experiences, can be dominant or recessive, and can be hidden from the narrator's awareness. For example, an action scheme can be present along with a trajectory of suffering but hidden from awareness. Therefore, biographical process structures allow for the simultaneity of multiple processes when analyzing life stories, thus providing a holistic and nuanced understanding of lived experience. Drawing on Anselm Strauss' research on terminally ill patients and their relationship to institutional processes, Fritz Schütze and Gerhard Riemann developed a theory of biographical and collective trajectories where they posited that aspects of social reality are not recognized by actors in their everyday life but can be analyzed by careful analysis of biography (Riemann and Schütze 1991). Schütze (1992) further argued that there can be collective trajectories. There were criticisms of whether a single case analysis was able to expand understanding about multiple cases and able to extend existing sociological theory (Apitzsch and Inowlocki 2000). The debate of generalizability from a single case analysis highlighted the fundamental relationship between theory and method and issues in communication and subjectivity, namely, if more than a reconstruction of intentionality within a given lifeworld was possible.

This debate was addressed by Schütze and other biographical researchers who emphasized the centrality of embeddedness of the biographical account in macro-level socio-historical conditions (Apitzsch and Inowlocki 2000). Schütze identified what he termed narrative constraints and cognitive figures as communicative narration schemes which enabled a deeper analysis of narratives to uncover biographical processes. Generalizability is thus made possible by examining substantive characteristics of narratives. The process of biographical analysis, especially of encountering unanticipated phenomena and of constant comparison of cases helps to generate new insights, makes the researcher especially attuned to the link between knowledge and the research process. Debates of realism versus idealism have also been placed against biographical research, and supporters of the biographical tradition responded by arguing that biographical research is based on a realist assumption that there is indeed a reality outside subjectivity which can be known (Apitzsch and Inowlocki 2000; Bertaux 2003). For example, Bertaux (2003) argued:

"Although life stories are undoubtedly subjective productions, they can be used as stepping stones to the construction of sociological descriptions and interpretations that come as close to objective sociological knowledge as is humanly possible. Moreover, life stories allow us to reintroduce into social research the dimension of time and the multiple temporalities of activities; this in itself is of extraordinary importance." (p. 41)

Bertaux (2003) defended the biographical approach and eloquently argued that although narratives are subjective, they still contain objective information. He even touched upon the quantitative versus qualitative research debate and advocated that life stories are more objective than survey measures and explained:

"If you limit your investigation to a given social phenomenon, and if you know how to combine life stories thus produced, you can move fast and deep into another cognitive direction; not that of statistical representativity, but that of in-depth description and understanding of how such a phenomenon takes place, and of when, where, why and with whom, according to which mechanisms and processes, norms and conflictual dynamics." (p. 43)

Bertaux strongly opposed the realist versus idealist debate considering it to be "absurd" while acknowledging the historical and constructionist aspects of social reality:

"I accept that the social world is also historical, and that the social-historical world, as an ongoing process or rather meta-process, rather than being a 'given' that needs to be studied and deciphered, gets constructed, co-constructed rather, reconstructed and transformed every minute by the activities and actions of people as agents." (p. 45)

Because Bertaux accepted the constructivist view, the implication from his arguments was that there must be a reality out there independent of our perceptions, and this reality can be at least partially observed and understood by research. Bertaux resolved the idealist versus realist debate in a powerful and concise argument:

"I can accept that I am not only an observer, but also a participant in this moving reality. But if you tell me there is no such reality, but only perceptions of it, representations of it, beliefs about it, I, as a sociologist, cannot follow, because it would mean the end of the sociological quest." (p. 45)

Bertaux (2003) thus powerfully asserted that there could be no interpretation if there was nothing or no reality to interpret and that we need a realist approach or else the discipline of sociology risks oblivion. Bertaux drew on Max Weber's and C. Wright Mills' views as co-constructionist and concluded:

> "It seems that the best way to understand a given set of phenomena would be to look for the processes that have produced them and reproduce them in (always slightly changed) forms. At the core of such a conception would lie a keen attention to the meanings alternative courses of actions have for actors. If taken seriously, this view leads to a capturing of the complexity of the real world, because social actions are also and always interactions. There is thus a potential convergence between Weber and interactionism; and what better definition of this potential point of convergence could be given than that provided by C. Wright Mills." (p. 47)

Therefore, biographical analysis is a valuable methodological approach which allows for a detailed analysis of life experiences rooted in historical context. The interplay between internal, individual experiences and social structural context is made visible in biographical analysis. Biographical analysis is thus a powerful tool for examining social reality at multiple levels of emergence. While narrative accounts are subjective, they are rooted in an objective reality. Immersion into narratives can help to generate new theoretical insights, further expanding our understanding of a given research topic and of social reality. Biographical analysis is a distinct approach which allows for multidimensionality in examining social phenomena, because when using this approach the dynamics of human action, social interaction, internal individual processes of change, personal and collective history, and social structural phenomena are all given attention and are analyzed in relation to one another.

Importantly, biographical analysis must be recognized as an approach with its own transatlantic and transcontinental history (Apitzsch and Inowlocki 2000). As Apitzsch and Inowlocki (2000) described, Fritz Schütze and Gerhard Riemann were influenced by American interpretive sociological concepts. Anselm Strauss influenced a number of German biographical researchers who in turn developed their own approaches to doing biographical research. Biographical research developed as an interchange of American and German influences on one another as the works of Alfred Schütz, George Simmel, and Karl Mannheim became especially influential on American research after WWII prior to influencing the field of qualitative-interpretative sociology in Europe. Apitzsch and Inowlocki (2000) outline how this mutual exchange between the United States and Germany unfolded over recent history and provide an interesting example of how Robert Ezra Park, who founded the Chicago School in American Sociology, traveled to Berlin, Germany where he was influenced by Simmel's work.

William Isaac Thomas and Florian Znaniecki (Thomas and Znaniecki 1927) are considered to be founders of biographical research within sociology as they used biographical documents in their seminal work *The Polish Peasant in Europe and America* (Apitzsch and Siouti 2007). Other prominent American researchers such as Hughes, Lindesmith, Becker, Strauss, and Garfinkel were influenced by the work of Simmel, Schütz, and Mannheim. This theoretical and methodological interchange between the United States and Germany was rooted in a context of migration as Jewish researchers from Germany and Austria were forced to migrate. Apitzsch and Inowlocki (2000) further described how this unique social context shaped the approach of biographical analysts who did not assume normality but instead focused on experiences in times of crisis and the emergence of a need for new social arrangements to prevent exclusion. With regard to the topic of this research, the focus on the prevention of exclusion and how people live through moments of crisis further emphasizes the advantage of using biographical analysis to understand the life experiences of PLWHA who face not only existential and mortality crises, but also social isolation and exclusion due to HIV stigma.

Biographical research was recognized as being important in order to understand people in their wholeness in order to examine otherwise hidden aspects of identity so that socially sensitive interventions could help to facilitate empowered self-views (Chamberlayne et al. 2000). Because my study focuses on HIV, a social status which is stigmatized, biographical analysis was especially useful in facilitating understanding and analysis of HIV as lived experience and for developing implications for empowerment of HIV identity. By drawing on the theoretical and methodological approach of Glaser and Strauss' (1965) grounded theory and carefully reconstructing each interviewee's narrative, an analysis of personal meaning and its link to action rooted in personal and social context was possible. Despite past critiques of the role of subjectivity and limits of generalizability, biographical research is a viable and fruitful approach which allows for the elaboration of concepts and processes based on the cases analyzed.

As Weber advocated in his Verstehen approach, an awareness of one's potential bias sensitizes the researcher to the research process and their own biases and how this can affect their research. Weber argued that by being socially sensitive we can effectively deal with bias (Weber 1949; 1978). Furthermore, the biographical analysis and constant comparative approach which involves constant revisions and editing, makes the researcher especially aware and especially attuned to the research process and their own personal bias and thus allows for an opportunity to acknowledge and overcome bias. Therefore, drawing on Weber's recommendations, we can begin to focus on the complementary nature of research techniques once we overcome outdated epistemological debates which can hinder collaborations between researchers from different methodological backgrounds due to heated refusals of alternate approaches to understanding social reality. This can encourage future research to integrate biographical analysis with other methodologies, which can be especially helpful in studies of health which is a major interdisciplinary research area.

2.2   Research Process of the Current Study

A biographical analysis would not have been possible without having narrative interviews. Narrative interviews were developed over time and based in research experience (Schütze 1983). As Riemann (2003) discussed, narrative interviews should involve the following characteristics: (1) a relationship of trust between interviewee and interviewer before and during the interview, (2) a generative question which elicits a narrative of the interviewee's involvement in a constellation of experiences and events that are relevant to the interviewee, (3) after the interviewee agrees to tell their narrative the narrative unfolds without any interruption by the interviewer so that the interviewee can reproduce their internal understanding of their experiences. The narrative continues until a coda which signals the end of the narrative. Interruption of the interviewee before the coda can disrupt the story line and thus make analysis more difficult. (4) A series of questions and answers which begins after the coda, that are based on the narrative and questions which elicit new material such as descriptions and theoretical-argumentational statements. Schütze (2007) argued that biographical analysis of narrative interviews is especially important when focusing on the life stories of those with chronic illness as he explained:

"Individuals in such a predicament react differently. Some try hard to return to an active attitude to life and attempt to take any imaginable road in order to find a new work position; others, on the contrary, feel totally paralysed and not able to take any initiative. The individual answer to the question whether at all and how to work with this predicament is very much influenced by the biographical preconditions of the life history of the individual. Many persons afflicted by chronic illness that results in unemployment and related problems did not learn how to deal with such a crisis situation. They might even have learnt *not to* deal with it at all, since in their childhood they had been discouraged to trust in themselves. They might not believe that they are capable of handling problems and conflicts in the family, with peers and in school or, later in life, to trust that they are able to handle difficult social relationships, work situations and depressing material conditions. But exactly this is the most important task in a rehabilitation situation: to activate oneself in order to become capable to shape one's own life. The central precondition of this is to do biographical work." (p. 2)

The concept of biographical work emphasizes how experiences of illness are rooted in biographical context and biographical aspects of the body, biographical time, and self-conceptions and allows for a focus on action (Corbin and Strauss 1988). Furthermore, as Schütze (2007) described, in the process of engaging in the narrative interview:

> "The autobiographical narrator or 'autobiographer' is retrospectively shaping her or his own biographical identity; but the task of the meaningful ordering of pieces of biography originally evolves from life historical experiences. She or he is the biography incumbent or the carrier of the history (or story) of her or his own life, and by telling it, or at least episodes of it, she or he is bestowing it with an elementary and systematic layer of meaningful order – offering a partial integration of chunks of meanings originally stemming from the formerly actually ongoing involvements within the concatenation of life-historical events themselves. The meaningful order of one's own life history has at its centre the unfolding of one's own biographical identity in relationship to the overall "gestalt" of concatenated and coexisting life historical processes." (p. 9)

Therefore, the narrative interviews allowed interviewees to communicate their biographies in relation to living with HIV in a personally meaningful form which was rooted in their own historical life experiences. Narratives unfolded without interruption as interviewees worked at making sense of their lives and to portray their experiences in the interview. As Schütze (2007) advised, narrative interviews must be analyzed in context and not as mere reflections of reality at face value. This can require the use of "pragmatic refraction" (Schütze 2005; Perleberg, Schütze and Heine 2006):

> "That naturally occurring verbal formulations should be analytically related to their contexts of experiential background, their contexts of production and use as well as to their contexts of later application, social function and meaningful overall (biographical or actional) structure. By consideration of the fivefold analytical embedding, i.e. pragmatic refraction, a more circumspect understanding of biographical work and grounding of autobiographical rendering becomes possible; even the understanding of experiences, which the autobiographical informant her- or himself recollects only dimly, does not understand correctly or doesn't understand at all, becomes possible." (Schütze 2007, p. 14)

When analyzing the narrative interviews I collected, I carefully related the interviews' textual content to these contextual factors in order to develop a deeper understanding of interviewee's narratives that was not based on the text on face value. Also, the issue of misrepresentation in narration was assumed to be unproblematic based on the formulation of Schütze (2007) that narrators rarely intentionally distort or lie and that fading out of certain parts of the narrative can be analyzed which can help to generate substantive insights. This was especially pronounced when analyzing the case of Walter (name changed) who was convinced that he did not have HIV and that he was instead an unwitting victim trapped in an experiment. By focusing on the construction of HIV as an experiment, a deeper understanding of Walter's story was made possible which generated new insights that helped to inform the analysis as it unfolded throughout Walter's narrative and the comparative analysis of the other cases.

Focusing on communicative schemes in the narratives, such as those of description, argumentation, and narration also guided the analysis. While multiple communicative schemes were present in the narratives, the dominant scheme of communication facilitated an analysis grounded in interviewee's telling of their stories. Communicative schemes also helped in the initial phases of the analysis when selecting the first case and a contrast case. For example, the case of Walter was selected due to his strong use of an argumentative communicative scheme as he actively strove to justify his belief that HIV was not real and was an experiment. The contrast case of Ana (named changed) was then selected as she engaged in more narrative and descriptive schemes of communication and accepted her HIV as real and also due to the involuntary and violent nature of her HIV infection. Communicative schemes as discussed by Schütze (2007) were important in the analytical process. The communicative schemes in the narratives were analyzed with a consideration of narrative constraints such as the constraint to: condense, go into details, and to close textual forms or gestalts (Schütze 1981; 1992; 2001).

Following Corbin and Strauss' (1990) guidelines for qualitative research procedures, I relied on theoretical sampling as I selected cases based on theoretical concepts and their dimensions, properties, and variations. The goal of this analysis was not the quantity of cases but the quality of analytical insights and the opportunities each case gave to further elaborate the analysis in a meaningful way. The process of conducting narrative interviews, transcription, and analysis was essential to the project and engaging in interviewing made me more aware of the interrelated nature of data collection and analysis (Corbin and Strauss 1990). Following the approach of grounded theory, concepts were analyzed as they emerged in the interviews concepts entered the analysis by:

> *"Repeatedly* being present in each interview, document, observation, in one form or another, or by being significantly absent (it should be there but isn't, thus we ask why). Having a concept demonstrate its relevance to the evolving theory (as a condition, action/ interaction, or consequence) is one way that grounded theory helps to guard against researcher bias. No matter how enamored the investigator may be of a particular concept, if it does not stand up to continued scrutiny through its repeated proven relevance to the phenomenon under question, it

must be discarded. The grounding of concepts in the reality of data, is what gives this method its
theory-observation congruence or compatibility." (Corbin and Strauss 1990, p. 420)

Therefore, although stigma and social support were concepts of interest driving
the inception of this study, these concepts were only included based upon their
emergence in the interviews and were modified as new dimensions and properties
emerged in the data. For example, social support shifted from an overarching
concept and was subsumed under broader biographical action schemes which
were emergent in the interviews. Stigma was a persistent aspect of interviewee's
stories and therefore remained a concept of interest. However, as unanticipated
phenomena such as the discussions of HIV as a secret and living a double life
emerged, the discussion of stigma shifted to a more interrelated and holistic
analysis of interviewee's experiences. Theoretical understanding and observation
shared compatibility and were intertwined in the research process. Theoretical
sampling of interviews helped to elaborate the analysis to the point of theoretical
saturation. Once saturation was reached the analysis continued to the next phase
of analyzing the Miami interviews.

Unfortunately, the data in Miami did not contain narrative interviews. Out of
this practical need, another need emerged. If this was to be a project that took
cultural context into account and framed the analysis in a comparative context
then interviews in two distinct locations met this need. Two samples allowed for
a cross-cultural comparison. The United States and Germany have different health
care systems which were essential in understanding illness experience. Issues of
racism and sexuality also emerged as important themes in both samples but were
unique to each location and rooted in location in personal and national history.
Such an analysis would not have been possible using only the Miami or
Frankfurt data in isolation.

Therefore, due to practical constraints, a cross-cultural comparison required a
comparison of two different types of interviews: narrative and topical interviews.
How did I compare these different types of interviews? I began by applying a
biographical analysis to the Frankfurt interviews. Working case by case, I
underwent an in-depth analysis of five exceptional cases. Each case was selected
based on the emergent themes and questions raised by the case before it. By
constantly comparing each case I was able to better understand participants'
narratives and to develop themes, processes, and a more detailed understanding
of the interviews. After these five cases had been analyzed in-depth and
compared, an additional three cases were analyzed with reports and integrated
case by case into the comparison. This process involved hundreds of pages of

analysis. The interrelatedness of life experience made conceptual decisions important at this stage. Deconstructing life experience and integrating it into a cohesive and meaningful whole to produce analytic insights was a challenging process that demanded constant revision and careful attention to conceptualization. Creating outlines of concepts and of the analysis helped to organize the analysis and was very helpful. After months of analysis, the analysis of the Frankfurt interviews was saturated and I moved on to the task of analyzing the Miami interviews.

I had begun a preliminary analysis of the Miami interviews approximately a year before and had to return to this data. I received a list of interesting cases and was advised to sort transcripts by length to select participants with longer interviews and more information in their transcripts. Some transcripts had multiple interviews (up to three) with case notes and notes from essays completed by participants over years of being involved in the research project. The list of interesting cases coincided with the cases with longer transcripts. I began to go through each transcript starting with the longest in the sample. An important difference in the types of interviews which shaped the data was the questions asked by the interviewer. Unlike the interviews I had conducted, the interviewer would ask questions throughout the interview which shaped the flow of interview and what topics were elaborated. However, by carefully rereading each transcript it was possible to reconstruct their story. Because the longer transcripts had case notes and multiple interviews it was possible to reconstruct their narratives. In the Frankfurt interviews, participants began their interviews with their diagnosis this allowed for a similarity in comparison because the first question the Miami participants were asked was about how they were living with HIV and often began with a discussion of HIV diagnosis. Based on the Frankfurt analysis, I used an outline to organize the Miami analysis. As with the Frankfurt analysis, it began with HIV diagnosis, the social context of diagnosis, and then went into reactions to diagnosis and experiences of stigma, agency, and other emergent themes. As I analyzed the Miami interviews, I constantly compared cases in the Miami sample to each other and also compared them to the Frankfurt sample. The use of a constant comparative approach facilitated the generation of new insights.

Time to reflect on analysis was also important. I also had to move in time between different phases of my project, as I tried to summarize my work I found myself drawing on my original ideas and attempting to integrate them with the analysis as it had developed. Biographical analysis required an extended period of time devoted to analysis and mental flexibility. A biographical approach challenged the researcher to rethink concepts and social processes and this challenge was a contribution of this methodology. Processes and conditions were understood and conceptualized from biographical perspective which helped to create a new understanding of social reality through lived experience.

2.3   Process, Context, and Conditions in Biographical Perspective

As an American researcher coming from a distinct scientific and sociological culture dominated by quantitative methodological approaches, the biographical analysis required an adaptation to this very different methodological approach. Rather than focusing on a statistical analysis, the analysis was textual and required a great deal of organization, theoretical revisions, and conceptual work. Relationships between phenomena and conceptualizations of concepts, processes, and conditions differ greatly between quantitative and qualitative traditions. In qualitative research, specifically following the approaches of researchers such as Fritz Schütze, Anselm Strauss, Juliet Corbin, and Gerhard Riemann processes are defined in much more nuanced ways than in quantitative research.

Processes are defined as more than statistically significant associations between variables; they are deeply embedded in personal and collective history and can overlap with other processes and conditions. Concepts become more fluid, process-based, and interrelated. Contextual conditions can be understood from the vantage point of a "conditional matrix" which emphasizes the complexity and interrelatedness of social reality and enabled a deeper and more nuanced analysis of my research questions than would be possible by relying on other methods. Developed by Corbin and Strauss (2007) and as discussed by Anselm Strauss (1993), a conditional matrix provides "ways of conceptualizing, discovering, and keeping track of conditions that bear on phenomenon – as defined by the researcher" (Strauss 1993, p. 60).

A conditional/consequential matrix is an analytical device used to stimulate thought regarding the range of possible conditions and consequences that can enter into context (Corbin and Strauss 2007, p. 229). Corbin and Strauss (2007) defined context as "The sets of conditions that give rise to problems or circumstances to which individuals respond by means of action/interaction/ emotions. Context arises out of sets of conditions ranging from the most macro to the micro" (p. 229). Process was understood as "Ongoing responses to problems or circumstances arising out of the context. Responses can take the form of action, interaction, or emotion. Responses can change as the situation changes" (Corbin and Strauss 2007, p. 229). Process is seen as more changeable and fluid. Corbin and Strauss (2007) described process as "The flow of action/interaction/emotions that occurs in response to events, situations, or problems. A change in structural conditions may call for adjustments in activities, interactions, and emotional responses. Actions/interactions/emotions may be strategic, routine, random, novel, automatic, and/or thoughtful" (p. 87). Using these conceptualizations of process, conditions, and context provides a more fluid and multi-level analytical perspective thus avoiding a static interpretation of narrative. Process is given agency by focusing on "processual ordering" of life experiences which "emphasizes the creative or constructive aspect of interaction the 'working at' and 'working out of' ordering in the face of inevitable contingencies" thus allowing for a deeper analysis of how order can be negotiated (Strauss 1993, p. 254). Conditions are conceptualized as necessary to processual ordering and as foundational components in processual ordering that contribute to social order and trajectories are seen as a broad concept for action which takes the dialectics of order to disorder and of stability to instability into account thus acknowledging the fluidity of social reality and it inherent changeable character (Strauss 1993, p. 257).

In contrast, quantitative methodology tends to focus on the concepts of mediator and moderator variables to understand process and conditions (Baron and Kenny 1986). A mediator is defined as a variable which specifies how or why a relationship occurs and is conceptualized as capturing the process linking two variables. A moderator is defined as a variable which affects the strength and or direction of a relationship between an independent and a dependent variable and is meant to assess the conditions under which a relationship is more or less pronounced (Baron and Kenny 1986). These definitions of mediator (process) and moderator (condition) allow for statistical analysis but compared to the definitions of process and conditions in qualitative methodology are not as comprehensive. Therefore, using a biographical perspective allowed for a much more nuanced understanding of social processes and conditions as they emerged in narratives of people living with HIV.

In order to more fully understand the life experiences of people with HIV, biographical processes and relevant contextual conditions are examined in the current study. Here, processes and conditions are defined in characteristically distinct ways in comparison to quantitative definitions of process and condition. The manner in which processes and conditions are conceptualized shapes our understanding of the social world and analysis of social reality. Biographical analysis allowed for a deep understanding of the unfolding of participants' lives with HIV which was grounded in their lifeworlds and allowed for a nuanced understanding of social processes and conditions and their embeddedness in individual and structural phenomena.

A single study can only examine so many statistical relationships between constructs. While quantitative research is extremely useful in demonstrating patterns and establishing evidence for relationships between social phenomena as measured with variables, the qualitative approach used here provides a more uninterrupted flow of experience as opposed to the snapshot of social reality quantitative studies provide. Using a biographical approach and applying the theoretical approaches to process, conditions, and context provided a nuanced and detailed understanding of social reality. A trade-off between the decision to use qualitative methodology as compared to quantitative methodology was the greater investment of time and corresponding financial resources and an extensive use of creative energy in analysis. With the efficiency-focused traditions of current American sociology, this may explain the lack of biographical analysis in the overall state of sociological research. However, the time and creativity expended on this methodology provided a more fluid and interrelated examination of how living with HIV was negotiated and how constraints were overcome to create new opportunities and of how personal growth was embedded in biography and social context. Biographical analysis is an extremely useful analytical approach which enables a unique analysis of the interplay between social structure and individual experience taking cultural context, history, and agency into consideration.

2.4   Centrality of Comparison in Generating New Insights

The research process which required a comparison of two samples and case-by-case comparison emphasized the centrality of comparison in generating new insights. As Corbin and Strauss (2007) posited, making comparisons was a fundamental aspect of the analytical process. The use of constant comparisons, as I compared case by case, allowed me to identify and distinguish themes from each other and to identify properties and dimensions of each theme.

Furthermore, the comparison of the Frankfurt and Miami samples allowed for additional insights to emerge which informed the analysis. The Frankfurt sample provided narrative interviews which were analyzed first. The structure of these interviews was open-ended and allowed interviewees to speak freely about their experiences. Follow-up questions were asked after the interview coda was expressed clearly that they had finished their narratives. Follow-up questions were based on subjects participants discussed in their narratives. The process of being on-site and being able to interview shaped process of analysis and allowed for a deeper involvement in the process as experiences by the interviewer and interaction with interviewees provided context to the analysis based on actual engagement with interviewees and also the opportunity to observe the social setting of their place of health care and the local context of Germany. The research design of the Miami involved semi-structured interviews which focused on spirituality and religion. Because the Miami interviews were not narrative, this required careful reading of all research materials with considerations of temporal ordering of life experiences and attention to multiple meanings and perspectives expressed at different times to create a coherent story. While narrative interviews in Miami would have been ideal, topical interviews were detailed, done at different points in time, and contained supplementary data which allowed for a reconstruction and understanding of the Miami sample's life experiences.

Both samples were of people living with HIV and thus they shared an important life experience. By comparing these samples the taken for granted assumptions of historical, socioeconomic, and cultural context were brought to attention. The comparison allowed an examination of whether what was important for one group of people in a specific location was also relevant for another group of people in a different context. This provided an opportunity to examine people living with HIV in different social contexts and how their experiences were related to this context. Also, the use of these two samples helped to provide social policy implications in regards to medical coverage of medication and of implementation of on-site support programs such as Helping Hand.

Practical considerations such as resources for research and the location and availability of research materials, shaped the research process and required multiple visits to both Frankfurt and Miami throughout the project's conception, implementation, and completion. However, traveling between both locations allowed for a unique experience of living in both cities which helped to facilitate reflections on the local context of both Miami and Frankfurt. Language also was a concern, only English-speaking patients could be interviewed in Frankfurt. Language proficiency was a limitation which was related to resources of funding and time. Despite this limitation, my sample included men and women both native to Germany and to other nations, with different ethnic backgrounds, sexual orientations, and time since their diagnosis.

By utilizing two samples, I was engaged in a dynamic research process which emphasized the local and national context of participant's experiences and how this was related to their biographies. The comparison between Miami and Frankfurt also facilitated an analysis which was informed by both the United States' and Germany's public policies of social security, immigration, and their unique histories. Without this comparison, the generation of new insights would have been restricted. Finally, by comparing these samples I was able to identify potential areas for change in policies that can affect HIV patients. In the next chapter, the research findings are presented.

3   Frankfurt am Main, Germany, and Miami, Florida, The United States of America: A Constant Comparative Case Analysis

In the following chapters the comparative analysis research and findings are discussed. First I provide the interview settings and case descriptions. Then, the findings of this study are organized into four parts. In Part 1, I discuss the conditions for the emergence of a trajectory of suffering. Next, in Part 2 biographical processes including processes of action and transformative processes are examined. Theoretical aspects of negotiating HIV such as disclosure and stigma are presented in Part 3. Finally, structural conditions related to negotiating HIV such as immigration and medical care social policies as experienced by participants are discussed. All names have been changed to ensure confidentiality.

3.1   Frankfurt am Main, Germany: Interview Setting and Case Overviews

In the summer of 2011 the interviews in Frankfurt took place on-site at an international HIV clinic. Ethics approval was obtained prior to initiating the interviews. After ethics approval was obtained I conducted the interviews from a small kitchen at the clinic and from different physicians' offices depending on the staff's schedules and preference. Physicians working at the clinic referred patients who were English-speaking. During this time, another doctoral student was present from a German university; she was a student of psychology. The clinic was open approximately twelve hours daily and I kept track each day of all of the physician appointments and their schedules.

The physicians and staff were aware of the purpose of my presence in the clinic and recognized and acted towards me as a student researcher and were helpful in referring patients. The interview context was characterized by friendly interactions between me and the medical staff. Although my role as a doctoral student in sociology was clear, in some cases, after the physicians potentially noticed the demeanor of some of the patients I had interviewed after our interviews, they referred some patients who appeared to be especially distressed and in need of therapeutic interaction. However, patients who had recently been diagnosed (less than one year since diagnosis) were not referred to me for interviews for ethical purposes. The patients were aware that I did not work at the clinic and of the purpose of their interviews. Some patients, particularly the older and more educated respondents expressed a concern for my research interests and a sensitivity to the topics mentioned in the consent process such as stigma and social support which guided my initial project. Some patients even made appointments and returned to have their interviews and thus expressed a desire to tell their story and an interest in my project. Patients often told that I was the only or first person to whom they had told their story. The interviews appeared to be a reflective process for interviewees. Overall, the interactions between myself and the patients were positive and the interview setting was characterized by mutual respect, privacy, and openness.

My analysis began with an in-depth analysis of the case of Walter. Walter was an exceptional case which was remarkable for many reasons. First, his interview was characterized by a predominately argumentative communicative scheme. Walter's argumentation made the suffering of HIV visible in a profound way as he continuously constructed his HIV as being unreal and expressed the belief that he was in an experiment. When I interviewed Walter, his attire consisted of headphones and a jacket to cover his work uniform, he was a security guard, but also was a musician. Walter's life involved participation in not only in different occupational spheres, but his HIV was kept completely separate from the rest of his life. Music emerged as an important part of his narrative and he seemed to be expressing his individuality and creativity by choosing to wear his jacket and headphones over his uniform. Walter was decidedly anti-conformist in his worldview and elaborated his beliefs in conspiracy theory in his argumentation. I selected Walter as the first case to analyze for these reasons. Also, because unanticipated themes such as debates of the nature of truth, reality, and entertainment emerged in his interview and because he emphasized historical racism in his argumentation, Walter's story presented a unique and exceptional case which drove the theoretical decision to analyze the second case of Rachel who served as a maximal contrast case to Walter.

The interview with Walter took place in a kitchen in the clinic. When I met Walter, I had an immediate feeling of familiarity since he was a fellow American (and as it later turned out, the only American I interviewed). I explained the interview and emphasized that I would not be asking questions. I explained this as we went over the consent form, he signed, and I told him I was turning on the recorder. The window was open and there were trains close-by. Walter suggested closing the window to improve the quality of the recording. His suggestion to close the window reminded me of a hip hop engineer I interviewed in Miami for a different project who had also in the beginning of his interview made sure the sound was good for the recording. Therefore, I was not surprised when Walter said he was a musician. Walter was very active, speaking passionately and powerfully. Walter repeatedly expressed his feeling that he was in an experiment. Walter told me many times his reason for this belief, he had unprotected sex for three years with a woman and she never contracted HIV and had an HIV-negative child with another man. Walter believed the government, the medical institution, or university had him in an experiment. He was a Black Muslim man who actively sought information and was politically engaged. Walter was defiant and expressed a strong will but was overwhelmed and confused by his HIV. He struggled in making sense of his HIV throughout his interview. Walter expressed a deep sense of betrayal and injustice for example he told:

> "All I can really say is um for some reason I feel betrayed (-) What I mean by betrayed is I feel (--) um (--) being that I'm at this big medical (--) ah school here (-) school cause there's a lot of students here (-) how are working on the grounds in the grounds (-) um for some reason I feel that I was (-) was (-) that I'm an experiment (-) for some reason. I can't tell you why I have that feeling (-) just a feeling I have within me (-) Um I just felt I'm an experiment (--) (--) and this is just to see what happens." [Transcript 1; lines 31-42[12]]

Walter could not articulate why, but deep within in him was the undeniable feeling that he was being betrayed, and his betrayal was related to his conception of HIV as an experiment. He described the clinic setting where there were students and it was a large medical facility. He could not say where this feeling that he was in an experiment came from. The feeling was "just within" him. Walter told the doctor that he did not think he had HIV. He had spoken to his

---

1   Transcripts not provided due to confidentiality concerns.
2   Transcription notation:
       (-) = get air with voice
       (--) = short pause in seconds
       [I: Hmm] = interventions by the interviewer
       bold = emphasis in speaking
       italics = softly spoken
       // = self-correction
       (uv) = incomprehensible text, guesses in brackets with question mark
       (laughs) non-verbal expressions

partner and his partner also did not think he had HIV. Walter was still in an active mode of thinking but he blended this subtly with elements of passivity because he felt betrayed and as if he was in an experiment, which was something out of his control. Walter maintained his argumentative mode but entered a trajectory of suffering as a victim of betrayal. He felt he had been placed in a situation against his will and could not define the reason for the existence of this experiment.

I made the analytical decision to contrast Walter's interview with the case of Rachel (name changed) an asylum seeker who had come to Germany from an African country. On the same day of the interview with Walter I interviewed Rachel. During my analysis, I chose Rachel's case as a maximal contrast to the case of Walter. I walked into the waiting room and Rachel was sitting with a cup of tea. We walked to the kitchen and I closed the door. I went over the consent form, she signed it, and I told her I was turning on the tape recorder. Rachel went directly into her story and within ten minutes she was crying, I looked around for tissues but there were none. I was concerned about her emotional state and asked Rachel if she was well and if she felt was able to continue. Rachel responded that she was well enough to continue. The reason Rachel was crying was because she was vividly describing how she had contracted HIV as a victim of sexual violence in a country ravaged by war:

> "Cause at the time I had no friends, I had no (--) I was sixteen years old (-) I had no friend (-) I never even thought about thinking about getting a boyfriend or that stuff also going to school, yeah (--) you know how it (voice strained) I don't know (begins to cry) um just came at night at home made us alone in the house our mom wasn't there (-) my big brother was also not there (--) (gets out tissues) and then one of them raped me and after they took my brother away with them they took him away so I remained at home I had nobody to talk to (-) My grandmother stays far relatively far away." [Transcript 2; lines 29-35]

Rachel discussed her difficulties in trusting others and only trusted doctors because she had to rely on them in order to get treatment. Having children was very important to Rachel and she had children after being diagnosed with HIV. While very different from Walter, both Rachel and Walter discussed their feelings of living a double life as being HIV-negative and as being HIV-positive. In contrast to Walter, Rachel had a reference group of HIV-positive people she could relate to in Helping Hand. Helping Hand helped Rachel to feel more comfortable going to use HIV services and reduced her fear of being seen seeking help.

Rachel displayed a very friendly, helpful, and kind demeanor. Rachel was an ideal contrast to Walter because she admitted her suffering and need for help in her struggles with HIV. Also, Rachel had accepted her HIV whereas Walter remained in denial of his HIV. Furthermore, unlike Walter, Rachel was a member of Helping Hand and the comparison between their cases allowed for an analysis of how involvement in this HIV support group could be related to group identification, the negotiation of living a "double life," and acceptance versus denial of HIV. Importantly, Rachel's country of origin and violent encounter with HIV at a young age were a contrast to Walter's experiences coming from the US and engaging in voluntary sex allowing for an examination of social context and contextual conditions in diagnosis and mode of transmission.

Next, the third, fourth, and fifth cases were selected to further elaborate emergent themes and their properties and to identify additional themes. The purpose of this analysis was to identify relevant themes as they emerged in the narratives in order to understand important issues in the lives of people living with HIV. All participants were interviewed on-site at a major HIV clinic in a large metropolitan city in Germany. First, a brief description of each case is provided, which includes demographic characteristics and observations from ethnographic protocols. Next, emergent themes are discussed. Full line-by-line case analyses were conducted for the first set (n=5) interviews. Subsequent interviews were analyzed using sequential reports. These interviews were selected based upon the process of theoretical sampling where cases were included based on their theoretical dimensions, properties, and variations (Corbin and Strauss 1990). Here I provide a brief overview over the additional cases of my analysis.

The third case was the story of Chris, an attractive gay man who was thirty one years old. His seemed to be of Hispanic or Middle Eastern descent. It was not clear if he was native to Germany or came from another country but he was very fluent in English. Chris was a teacher but had worked in the past at a gay sex shop. He went directly into his story about his diagnosis and his experiences afterwards, he was well-spoken and thoughtful.

The forth case was that of Arthur, a white, European, middle-aged Gay man native to Germany. Arthur was diagnosed in the 1990s. He discussed his past lifestyle as risky and involving "sex, drugs, and rock and roll." Arthur had a successful career and was retired at the time of the interview. The fifth case was Sarah, another patient living with HIV for decades. She was a middle-aged Turkish woman, widowed, with two sons, and self-employed. Sarah had been living with HIV for twenty years.

The sixth case was Alice, an African woman, in her adult years (she appeared to be in her early thirties), married with children. She was also diagnosed with Tuberculosis which was successfully treated after one year. Nina was a member of Helping Hand. The seventh case was George, a white, European, middle-aged gay man. George had a near-death experience and was first misdiagnosed with cancer. He was living with HIV for one year and was married to his gay partner of twenty years.

The eighth case was David, a gay African man in his adult years who lived in Germany since the age of seven. David had been living with HIV for three years and was a member of Helping Hand. His HIV status was revealed by a local newspaper covering his involvement in providing HIV information to African communities in Frankfurt. He was employed and educated with a good income.

Following the approach of Schütze (1983), which has more recently been described by Apitzsch and Siouti (2007), I began with a sequential case analysis of the first case of Walter. The analysis of the first case involved a formal textual analysis, where I transcribed the interview and segmented the interview into thematic segments. Next I engaged in a structural description of the interview segments in order to identify biographical structural processes. The structural description was completed in sequential order (Riemann 2003). The structural description helped me to describe and analyze the interview using a line by line analysis to reconstruct the meaning of the narrative. Next I used analytical abstraction to identify the overall the Gestalt of the interview which allowed me to develop themes and their properties and dimensions. I then compared and contrasted the case analyses of Walter and Rachel in order to generate additional theoretical insights. The additional cases were analyzed sequentially and substantively and were included case by case in a constant comparative analysis to identify additional themes and to elaborate emergent themes.

3.2   Miami, Florida, the United States of America: Research Setting and Case Overviews

The Miami interviews took place in a different research setting than the interviews in Frankfurt. Importantly, I did not conduct the interviews in Miami. The parent study was conducted in Miami, Florida as part of a longitudinal study of stress and coping with HIV (Ironson et al. 2005). Subsequent analysis of the qualitative data and substudies on spiritual Transformation and Spiritual Coping were conducted by both Drs. Ironson and Kremer. Dr. Gail Ironson is an

American researcher who is both a physician and a health psychologist working as a professor at the University of Miami where she runs the "Positive Survivor's Research Center." Participants in her study were a paid volunteer sample and were recruited through physician offices, specialty clinics, hospitals, service organizations, and advertisements newspapers and gay publications and were compensated 50USD per visit in their earlier studies and were compensated 75USD in their later studies. Institutional Review Board (IRB) approval was obtained and participants consented to the use of their de-identified data.

The participants were interviewed every six months at the research center and also provided blood, urine, and saliva samples, completed questionnaires, and wrote essays. Most of the interviews were completed by the principal investigator's staff and were often transcribed by her students. The interviews were topical and interviewees were asked about their spirituality and HIV as a life-changing event. I had worked as a research assistant using this data at this center years ago. Dr. Heidemarie Kremer was involved in the development of my doctoral dissertation and, with her experience in the American and German academic systems, served as an advisor to my doctoral dissertation and a liaison between the University of Miami and Goethe University. Also, during the completion of this study I worked with Dr. Gail Ironson and Dr. Heidemarie Kremer as an analyst for two projects.

During this time we communicated between three countries: the US, Germany, and Indonesia. Dr. Heidemarie Kremer and I met in Frankfurt, Berlin, and Köln for brief meetings but during my studies she was based in Bali, Indonesia. I was advised to go through their interview transcripts beginning with the longest transcripts because these had more complete data. I was also given a list of interesting cases by Dr. Heidemarie Kremer and based on her recommendations and the data available I selected cases to analyze. These interview transcripts contained multiple interviews, essay excerpts, and case notes. The use of different research materials was challenging but integral to the possibility of making a cross-national comparison.

The analysis of the Miami interviews was informed by the analysis of the Frankfurt interviews. Using theoretical sampling, I made the analytical decision to include six cases in the Miami data. These cases were analyzed and presented in my doctoral work which I defended with Dr. Heidemarie Kremer as a third member of my dissertation committee. However, upon my return to the United States and subsequent meetings with both Dr. Gail Ironson and Dr. Heidemarie Kremer concerns regarding the confidentiality and rights of their interviewees surfaced. The US has a unique research context where there are deep seated concerns over ethics and intellectual property. Dr. Gail Ironson's research project was approved by the Institutional Review Board (IRB) but due to the novel integration of data sources and the different academic systems in Germany and the U.S. the dissemination of research findings was undergone in an ambiguous context. Therefore, in order to ensure the confidentiality of their interviewees, I removed their stories and all quoted materials from the Miami data in this manuscript. Future research involving international, collaborative efforts could be improved by developing clear, coordinated standards of evaluation and research protocols between researchers, institutions, and participants. Despite this restriction in dissemination, in this manuscript I present the findings of my comparative analysis to the best of my ability without identifying participants. The concerns surrounding the issue of confidentiality in HIV research appeared to reflect the fear of stigma and discrimination of revealing HIV status. HIV stigma can result in the loss of professional careers, intimate partnerships, and social relationships. The stigma and fear surrounding disclosure of HIV manifested in the form of a restriction in the dissemination of my research findings.

This analysis does not introduce each case sequentially in the order of their inclusion. Instead each case enters the analysis based on the theoretical dimensions which emerged in the analysis. Because the Miami data narratives could not be presented only the analysis presented in completely de-identified and generalized form remains. All names have been changed to maintain anonymity.

3.3   Part 1: Conditions for Trajectory of Suffering Potential

3.3.1   Circumstances and Social Context of HIV Diagnosis
as Conditions for the Emergence of Trajectory of Suffering

Importantly, all participants began their narratives with the moment of their diagnosis or the circumstances in their initial encounters with HIV regardless of their age, race/ethnicity, gender, and time since diagnosis. This highlights the importance of HIV diagnosis in the unfolding of their biographical trajectories. A trajectory of suffering is one type of biographical process, which as discussed in the introduction chapter involves a growing sense of a loss of control over one's life circumstances and feelings of incomprehensibility and confusion over meaning in one's life. A trajectory of suffering is distinct from other conceptualizations of trajectory such as that of the life course perspective which defines a trajectory as a life course concept which involves sequences of roles and experiences and transitions of changes in states or roles (Elder 1996). Although trajectory in life course theory is grounded in historical experience, this conceptualization differs from the concept of "trajectory of suffering" (Riemann and Schütze 1991), where trajectory of suffering is seen as more than roles and experiences in sequence and transitions in states or roles and involves a loss of control over one's life that is related to structural processes structured by conditional chains of events. This chain of events cannot be avoided and is characterized by a growing sense of a loss of control and is conceptualized as a biographical process which has conditions of emergence, phases, and ways out. Biographical processes are distinct but can overlap. Trajectory in the life course theory is subsumed under broader social pathways whereas trajectory of suffering in biographical analysis is an analytical concept used to understand disorderly social processes in biography.

HIV diagnosis had the potential seeds of an emergence of a trajectory of suffering. Because there are numerous biographical processes including process structures of action, a trajectory of suffering involves an ongoing tension and the possibility of an exit into other biographical processes. These other processes will be discussed further in later chapters. In regards to the emergence of a trajectory of suffering, certain conditions emerged as related to undergoing a trajectory of suffering. The social context and conditions of HIV diagnosis emerged as important contextual conditions related to biographical process. Importantly, participants discussed their HIV diagnosis by bringing in the social and personal contexts of their diagnosis in a very descriptive, vivid way. For example, Rachel's description of how she contracted HIV through involuntary sexual contact in an area plagued by military conflict and violence was charged with emotional upset and imagery.

Rachel visited the doctor after being raped by soldiers in her home and discovered she was pregnant. Rachel decided to have an abortion because of the traumatic circumstances surrounding the child's conception. This occurred in Rachel's African country of origin in a small village where violence and poverty were a fundamental aspect of the socio-cultural context. Despite the trauma of being a victim of sexual violence and having an abortion, Rachel framed her diagnosis in a positive way. She felt that her diagnosis helped her because if she had not been diagnosed she felt she could have died. In contrast, Walter who had visited the doctor for the treatment of cirrhosis described his diagnosis in a negative way. The physician asked Walter during that visit if he consented to a HIV test and about two weeks later he was called into the office and told he had HIV.

Walter felt extremely shocked and compared his diagnosis to a punch in the face and to a heavy blow. Walter brought in dialogue suggesting that this was a critical moment in his narrative. Walter felt deeply betrayed and that his life had been destroyed. The metaphor of a punch to the face and a heavy blow indicate not only the emotional context of his diagnosis but his conceptions of HIV from the beginning of his life with HIV. The metaphor of a physical attack suggests an element of violence and pain in his diagnosis. Walter's violent and metaphorical comparison to his diagnosis to a physical attack suggests that although this was an emotional and painful moment, he framed his pain in a masculine manner rather than admitting emotional pain in this critical moment in his narrative.

The terms employed to describe initial encounters with HIV can be representative of the social meaning ascribed to HIV by the narrators. The terms "heavy blow" and "confronted with" suggest that feelings of threat and danger were an element of the emotional context of HIV diagnosis. Participants' descriptions of HIV diagnosis as a "shock" and feeling as if they were "dreaming" indicated the drastic shift in orientation to the world due to being thrown into a new identity as someone with HIV. HIV diagnosis involved being faced with what was described as a perceived initial death sentence and which posed an imminent threat to mortality.

HIV diagnosis presented an existential dilemma where participants were thrown into circumstances beyond their control and where they reported feelings of distress, unreality, and incomprehensibility of their new reality of having HIV. Importantly, while HIV diagnosis presented itself as a condition for the beginning of a trajectory of suffering, later biographical processes, under certain conditions, allowed participants to escape their trajectory of suffering and to regain control over their lives. Escaping the trajectory of suffering involved processes of making sense of HIV, which was facilitated by the availability of support, resources, and information about HIV and biographical work aimed at integrating an HIV-positive identity to existing self-conceptions. These processes of coming to terms with HIV were rooted in participants' life experiences and histories.

The circumstances in participants' personal histories shaped how their diagnoses were experienced and contributed to reactions to diagnosis. Specifically, mode of HIV transmission, health status, and socio-cultural context emerged as conditions affecting the experience of HIV diagnosis and as being related to biographical processes. For example, Rachel was in poor health, a victim of sexual violence, and in need of medical treatment. In contrast, Walter was in good health, had no symptoms, and visited the doctor only for the treatment of a skin condition. Perhaps Rachel was more helpless in her situation from the moment she contracted HIV, as suggested by her feeling that if she had not been diagnosed she could have died. Despite powerlessness and experiencing violence, isolation, and rejection Rachel was positive about her diagnosis. Rachel accepted her HIV diagnosis and treatment as being essential to her survival. Rachel was close to death and seriously ill when she was diagnosed as a teenager, which suggests that health status at the moment of diagnosis can be an important factor shaping acceptance of illness and treatment. The comparison of Rachel and Walter demonstrated how sociocultural context, health status, and mode of transmission emerged as a condition shaping the experience of HIV diagnosis.

There were contextual differences between Rachel and Walter's experiences when they contracted HIV. Their positions in society were distinct. For example, unlike Walter, Rachel was defenseless in a war situation in a nation with limited economic resources and health care where she was victimized and socially isolated. In contrast, Walter contracted HIV through voluntary sexual contact in a context of living in a developed and wealthy nation with advanced medical care. However, despite the wealth and health care in the United States, the high levels of inequality and racism in the United States problematized Walter's experiences.

When Walter was diagnosed he felt healthy and was already an adult. Interestingly, he could not recall the moment or circumstances of his HIV infection. For Walter, the origins of HIV were unclear and because he had no health impairments the existence of HIV was doubted. An understanding of the cause of HIV transmission was reported as important to participants' coping with HIV. This supports the conceptualization of coping with HIV as involving biographical work to deal with HIV as a trajectory of suffering because as Riemann and Schütze (1991) argued a feature of a trajectory of suffering involves:

> "The sources and features of the powerful outer forces are at least partially unknown, experienced as inconceivable, they gain even more power in the eyes of the sufferer. At least in the beginning the person cannot plan counteractivities because she or he doesn't know exactly enough what is going on. A sense of fate and generalized feeling of uncertainty darkens the life horizon of the person." (p. 343)

While not deterministic, the context of transmission may set the stage for the unfolding of a life trajectory with HIV, shaping the context of diagnosis, which in turn can have cataclysmic effects on the sequence and experiences after diagnosis. This process itself involves processes and conditions which shape each other over time, and so biographical analysis was especially useful in examining coping responses to HIV as a dynamic process.

My comparison of Walter and Rachel drove the analytical decision to include Chris as a third case in this comparison. Chris and Walter were similar in regards to their age, time since diagnosis, having voluntary sex as their mode of HIV transmission, and both felt that they were healthy. However, unlike Walter, Chris was a gay man and contacted HIV through a threesome which he clearly identified as the cause of his HIV. Similar to Rachel, Chris went directly into his story about his diagnosis and his experiences with HIV. Importantly, Chris and Rachel both accepted their HIV but Chris was not a member of Helping Hand. The strong emphasis of love and appearance in interaction also drove the decision to include Chris in the analysis. Unlike Walter, Chris identified the context and cause of his HIV diagnosis and was later able to accept his HIV diagnosis. The identification of a clear cause of HIV infection facilitated greater acceptance of HIV. Also, HIV diagnosis presented a dilemma in managing intimate relationships. The negotiation of intimate relationships was problematic when sexual partners were HIV-negative. Chris' HIV diagnosis introduced a moment of crisis where he struggled with a new definition of himself as a potential threat or danger to his partner's health and had to face the decision to disclose his HIV status and to risk losing his partner.

Importantly, fundamental questions of "Where did this come from?" "How did I come in touch with HIV?" and "Why me?" presented major dilemmas for participants upon their HIV diagnosis. This questioning can be conceptualized as part of a process in the beginning phases of HIV as a trajectory of suffering. For example, Walter described:

> "My question is 'Why me?' Why […] I have this (-) this (-) this (-) this excuse my language, my derogatory language, this fucking virus? Why? And how? And how come nobody else is infected that I've been in contact with but I'm infected? How? How?" [Transcript 1; line 284-290]

The search for meaning and the sense of losing a grasp of reality was further elaborated by Walter:

> "I don't know I'm kinda stuck in limbo as to where, when, how, who, and what, but I feel I don't care what nobody tells me, I don't care what kinda psychologist, psychiatrist, I don't give a fuck what you do nobody can tell me that this (-) can take this aggression away from me cause this is (-) I don't care (-) this is deliberately done." [Transcript 1; lines 594-599]

Other participants also reported struggles with the question of "Why me?" but Walter's case clearly demonstrated the struggle in meaning making of HIV as he asked:

> "I need to know where did this (voice rises to questioning tone) (-) Why was it AIDS first then HIV? Why wasn't it HIV and then AIDS? First it was AIDS then HIV. Why? You know? Why wasn't it vice versa? Cause HIV turns into AIDS but how do we become aware of it? First it was AIDS, then it was broken down to the virus of HIV, how is that? (--) Makes no sense" [Transcript 1; lines 942-952]

Walter's communicative scheme was argumentative as he struggled with making sense of his diagnosis. His construction of the meaning of HIV was related to the social context of his diagnosis. One aspect of the context of Walter's diagnosis was the inability to identify the cause of his HIV infection. Being able to clearly identify the cause of HIV infection helped other participants to makes sense of their diagnosis.

Rachel began by telling where she was from and then moved on to explain her reason for coming to Germany. Her mother first moved to Germany before Rachel's father died. After her father's death, Rachel described that there had been many "critical problems" including the kidnapping of her older brother in her home in a small village in her African country of origin. Rachel continued her story, after her mother left, Rachel was alone. Rachel then described how the soldiers came into her home and sexually victimized her when she was a virgin and sixteen years old. The circumstances of her encounter with HIV were characterized by powerlessness and isolation. Rachel was young, alone, and a victim of sexual violence. This was a very emotional part of her narrative she began to cry as she told her story. After the soldiers took Rachel's brother she remained alone at home with no one to talk to. The socio-cultural context of Rachel's cause of HIV infection was characterized by violence, poor medical care, and her own personal isolation.

Similar to Rachel, Chris went directly into his diagnosis and brought in the social context of this episode as he was diagnosed around the same time a year before the interview and he was with his ex-boyfriend of three and a half years who also accompanied him to the clinic on the day of our interview. Chris began his narrative by starting with his diagnosis and discussed his intimate relationships and the context of the moment when he knew he has HIV as he described:

"I met someone else last year [...] and um fell in love over again because I was looking for someone more emotional in a relationship and we still had like (-) we still spoke and so after a couple of months he called me like (-) I was like at a friend's and I had like 18 miss calls on my phone and already could tell that something was going on (-) something wasn't ok (-) so I called him back. (-) and he was just crying and he said that um that he's HIV-positive (-) so in that moment I just helped a friend he was in a clinic he was having mental issues so he asked if we could go get him out and take care of him so we (-) yeah I had that friend with me in the car and I was on the phone just driving off as he tells me that he's HIV-positive (-) so I automatically knew (-) that means I'm positive too (-) there's no way I can be negative (-) so I was like (-) first of all like I was really (--) it was just like a dream I couldn't focus (-) I was just driving (--) I like (--) subconsciously probably was paying attention to all the um traffic but I was kinda really out of my body." [Transcript 3; lines 9-21]

This moment was contextualized in biographical experience and the context of social relationships. Chris knew that he must also have HIV. Upon this discovery, Chris felt that moment was "just like a dream." This experience was surreal and Chris was in shock. Shock upon diagnosis was reported by other participants. The shock at diagnosis indicated a confrontation with an existential dilemma that threatened conceptions of the self, intimate relationships, and health. HIV diagnosis required the biographical process of "contextualizing" HIV into participant's biographies (Strauss 1993). The process of coming to terms with HIV can unfold over time and those living with HIV for many years provided a contrast to newly diagnosed patients. Therefore, time since diagnosis emerged as a condition which affected coping with HIV.

Because social context of diagnosis and time since diagnosis emerged as important parts of HIV experience I made the analytical decision to include Arthur as the forth case. Unlike the first three cases, Arthur was middle aged and had lived with HIV for decades. Arthur framed his HIV diagnosis in the social context of the decade when he was diagnosed. The 1980s were a time characterized by less developed HIV medication, a lack of medical and public understanding of HIV, and where death was described as the expected outcome of having HIV when death from AIDS was rampant. Similar to Chris, Arthur was a gay man who accepted his diagnosis but he had experienced generational change in the views of gays and of HIV. Another reason for the inclusion of Arthur in this analysis was his emphasis on his success in his career in a well-paid, prestigious position that allowed him to retire at an early age. Arthur's emphasis on the importance of professional standing and economic resources made him a unique case.

Arthur did not discuss having any health problems at the time of his diagnosis, but did explain that his access to clinical trials and health care helped him to adjust to his HIV and to survive. Arthur began his narrative by providing his name, age, sexual orientation, race, and gender. He framed the term "gay white man" as a term which Americans would use to describe him. He grouped his sexual orientation, race, and gender together but kept his name and age separate from these other social characteristics as he described himself. Arthur explained that he had been gay for his entire life, emphasizing that his identity as a gay man has been a long-term identity and was an important aspect of his definition of self.

Arthur continued directly to describe the social context of his diagnosis. Arthur contextualized his HIV diagnosis by explaining his age at the time of diagnosis, the amount of time that has passed since then, and the historical decade of the 1980s a time when HIV was a new epidemic and medical treatment had not yet sufficiently developed. Arthur initially felt that his HIV diagnosis was a death sentence and that he only had a few more years to live. Over two decades after his HIV diagnosis, Arthur still recalled the shock of his diagnosis. This is similar to the other participants who all described feelings of shock at the moment of HIV diagnosis. This suggests that the moment of HIV diagnosis remains a salient moment even after years spent living with HIV.

After including Arthur's case in the comparison, I made the analytical decision to include Sarah as the fifth case. Similar to Arthur, Sarah had been living with HIV for decades and this allowed for a comparison of those who were living with HIV for a long period of time, diagnosed in a different generational and social context, and in a later stage in their life course. Sarah was an exceptional case for many reasons. Similar to Arthur she was a professional and appeared to be successful as she worked independently. However, Sarah was infected with HIV by her deceased husband and this was a distinct mode of transmission from the other cases. Sarah also already had her children when she was diagnosed and she emphasized the importance of caring for her children in the context of being diagnosed with HIV.

Distinct from the other cases, Sarah underwent psychoanalysis for years and she discussed this as central to her process of taking action in her narrative. Both Arthur and Sarah discussed having other health problems and this was important to examine in the context of HIV. Similar to Arthur, Sarah did not describe having other health problems when she was diagnosed with HIV. The HIV diagnosis of Sarah's husband lead Sarah to her own HIV testing and diagnosis. Similar to Arthur, Sarah had been living with HIV for many years and discussed the social context of her HIV back in the 1990s. Sarah went directly into the beginning of her life with HIV in her interview as she explained how she and her husband were both ill in the early 1990s. Sarah's husband became severely ill and was hospitalized here at the hospital which is where Sarah first encountered her new life with HIV. Similar to the other cases, Sarah described her HIV diagnosis as a drastic change in her life:

> "Well that was a big shock of course (-) immediately I got the children tested and they were ok (-) and uh after that I had myself then tested (-) probably I was so scared and frightened see? Uh after the first I didn't go to get the results (-) I just didn't (-) you just start to ignore right?" [Transcript 5; lines 17-31]

Sarah explained the emotional shock she experienced at her discovery of her husband having HIV. The emotional context of Sarah's diagnosis involved a consideration of her children's well-being, her own shock at the discovery of her husband's HIV, and a deep fear of the possibility that she also had HIV. Sarah's fear of HIV lead her to wait to get her results despite the imminent and perceived threat of HIV, which suggests that her fear lead her to a moment of denial and distance from this confrontation with HIV. She explained:

> "I didn't know anything (-) I mean he was in the neurological department and uh they call me for uh a conversation (-) for an interview and the first thing the doctor said to me '**Do you know that your husband has HIV**?'" [Transcript 5; lines 7-12]

This moment appeared to be critical as Sarah described how the doctor told her about her husband's HIV status. The doctor did not tell her, rather he asked her about her HIV. Her discovery of HIV was presented to her in the form of a question. Did she know that her husband had HIV? This question was presented clearly and with a notable change in her tone of voice to emphasize the enormity of this question. In this moment Sarah's world was fundamentally altered. This was the beginning of her life with HIV. She framed this experience in the social context of the 1990s:

> "Well you heard something here and there about it (-) you just knew it's something very dangerous uh ah nothing besides that (-) that was (-) that was the way I was confronted with that." [Transcript 5; lines 12-15]

It was the early 1990s, twenty years ago when Sarah first encountered HIV, a time when information about HIV was not as widespread as today. Sarah's experiences, as reported in the interview, suggested that HIV remains a taboo subject in public discourse in Germany as she told about her secret life with HIV.

When she was first confronted with the reality of HIV, the only aspect of HIV which Sarah was aware of was the dangerousness of HIV. Her encounter with HIV was described as a confrontation which suggests that this was a moment that was against her will and which she had to face and fight.

Due to the importance of cultural context in the descriptions of the Frankfurt sample of their life experiences with HIV, a cross-cultural comparison to interviews conducted with participants in Miami was utilized. Similar to the German sample, participants in Miami vividly recalled their HIV diagnosis. HIV diagnosis was described as a major event in their lives and participants framed their diagnosis in social context. HIV was experienced as a catalyst for major life changes and biographical work. Biographical processes of both suffering and of action unfolded overtime and were deeply tied to social context of diagnosis and life conditions of participants. Having HIV forced people to face the reality of their mortality by facing their own illness and the deaths of their loved ones. The pain and sense displacement of having to adapt to a new life with HIV was an emergent theme in both the Miami and Frankfurt samples. Reactions to HIV diagnosis were embedded in participants' personal histories. HIV can become a part of awareness prior to diagnosis due to personal experiences. Conceptions of HIV prior to diagnosis affected how HIV diagnosis was experienced. Involvement with the HIV community before HIV infection was an important aspect of personal history related to conceptions of HIV. The social context of sudden and rampant death in the 1980s and 1990s was emphasized by those living with HIV for many years.

Initial encounters with HIV were described as surreal. In these moments, reality was rendered strange and unbound by the external flow of time. Consistent with a phenomenological perspective, the intimate relationship between consciousness, time, and memory was explicit as HIV entered participants' awareness and fundamentally changed their life worlds in moments described as outside of time, characterized by feelings of unreality, with dream-like qualities that evaded memory (Bergson 1922; Husserl 1964; Husserl and Brough 1991).

A context of death and fear was described by participants who were diagnosed in the 1980s and 1990s. Some participants described living a risky lifestyle where HIV was always a risk. Mode of HIV transmission shaped the reaction to diagnosis in both samples. In the context of an overall risky lifestyle and when mode of transmission was perceived as a result of voluntary behavior, HIV was not described as being as shocking and was more easily accepted. This context of death and fear shaped experiences of not only diagnosis but of HIV disclosure. Participants emphasized the social pressures of regulating and masking their emotional struggles and identity. Deaths of loved ones were common. For interviewees, concerns over their parents' health and additional trauma of having parents pass away were stressful, exacerbating an already difficult life situation. Participants also discussed having friends die of AIDS and how the deaths of others due to AIDS reminded them of their own HIV status and mortality. Dealing with the loss and the illness of loved ones while being sick themselves, participants had to come to terms with both their own HIV and the illness and deaths of others.

Women in both samples emphasized their concern for their children and often discussed issues related to having HIV and managing their pregnancy in order to as to prevent HIV transmission to their children. Caretaking was an important role for these women. Relations of care were related to their giving compassionate love and taking action to survive and make positive life changes to enhance their health. Positive life changes included the cessation of drug use and overall risky lifestyles and the strengthening their faith in themselves and the spiritual. Relations of care were not specific to only women but were also important to the men interviewed in both samples.

Despite the initial shock and painful experiences of rejection that were encountered upon diagnosis and disclosure of HIV status, participants were able to overcome the challenge of HIV. In a prior study of people living with HIV, a substantial number or those reporting that HIV as a negative turning point in their lives also report experiencing a secondary positive life change (Kremer et al. 2009). Cessation of drug use and other risky health behaviors can occur after HIV diagnosis. Participants in both samples reported a level of acceptance and awareness of HIV if they attributed the cause of HIV to their own voluntary behavior. However, when mode of transmission was viewed as outside their control, for example being due to an unfaithful partner or to unforeseen causes, acceptance of HIV required more time and effort. In this context, denial at initial diagnosis and shock were common and difficulties integrating HIV into biography were heightened. Therefore, the socio-cultural context of HIV diagnosis and mode of HIV transmission served as conditions for biographical coping. Mode of transmission in the Miami sample was reported as being due to risky sexual behavior or prior drug use. However, infidelity by a partner was reported as a cause of HIV infection. Therefore, infection can occur in a context of what seems to be a safe environment due to the seeming sexual security of a relationship.

The importance of time since diagnosis and the temporal dimension of living with HIV were emphasized by participants. Although initial reactions to HIV involved shock, denial, and fear of death participants learned to negotiate their HIV over time and to make healthy, productive changes to help them to live with HIV. HIV diagnosis can serve as a "reality check," motivating people to stop risky lifestyles. However, HIV diagnosis cannot be divorced from the lifeworlds of participants because constellations of events coalesced to help facilitate life change. HIV was not experienced in a social vacuum and was deeply rooted in personal life situation, history, and social context. For some participants change was abrupt or experienced as sudden, whereas for others, change was viewed as something that needed to be maintained constantly over time or which was a gradual process.

Reconciling spiritual or religious conflicts emerged as an important aspect of coming to terms with HIV over time. Religious stigma and conflicts of identity and conceptions of sin and free will emerged in the Miami interviews. The relationship between religious conceptions of sin and sexuality were also discussed by Arthur in the Frankfurt sample. Religious issues may have been emphasized more in the Miami sample due to the interview questions focusing on spirituality and religion. When participants possessed an additional deviant status such as that of drug addiction, being gay or criminal behavior the issues of coming to terms and reintegrating religious doctrines and developing their spirituality were important in accepting HIV and themselves. Interestingly, while some participants in Frankfurt reported histories of drug use and risky lifestyles, explicit reports of drug use and involvement in deviance and criminal behavior were more common among the Miami sample. Also, poverty and issues in obtaining health care and medication were discussed more often among the Miami sample. Life change was often related to a constellation of events and stressors such as having HIV and living in poverty.

Furthermore, participants wrestled with the question of "Why me?" as they struggled to make sense of their HIV. When wrestling with this question, participants in both the Miami and Frankfurt samples discussed the importance of the truth, knowledge, identity as they made sense of HIV. Other participants reported the belief that they had gotten HIV in order to help others or to grow. Therefore, themes of HIV as a means of personal growth and transformation and as a means to help others and to become more compassionate emerged. Despite initial struggles with making sense of HIV, participants in both samples reported positive outcomes. Therefore, it is critical to more fully understand what conditions are conducive to positive outcomes among people living with HIV. Understanding exceptional cases of transformative change can help develop a more systematic model of how people living in a context of disadvantage and adversity can overcome stressful events and go on to lead meaningful and productive lives.

Transformative change can be related to the schemes of meaning people construct regarding the etiology of their infection. Importantly, participants came to terms with their HIV diagnosis by finding a deeper meaning and purpose for their HIV beyond the immediate social context of their infection. This process of meaning making and negotiating HIV into biography appeared to be rooted in time as participants reflected back on their experiences and described how they negotiated HIV over time. Initial feelings of shock, pain, and denial eventually gave way to acceptance and productive approaches to living with HIV. The initial negative life experience of HIV diagnosis was often followed by positive life change and life change was intertwined with other life experiences, which coalesced and then crystallized in participants' awareness that they could act to improve their lives. This crystallization of the possibility for a better life was an awareness of agency that preceded taking action, thus facilitating empowerment and illuminating resiliency in the face of adversity. This awareness occurred through various biographical process structures. Some of these processes were identified in the Frankfurt sample such as compassionate love and relationships of care but new processes emerged in the Miami interviews and are discussed in the section on biographical process structures.

3.3.2   Health Status at Diagnosis and Personal Histories of Medical Treatment

Another element of social context that emerged as a condition affecting processes of making sense of HIV was health status at time of diagnosis. For some participants, other health problems lead to their diagnosis. Walter came to the hospital due to skin problems with cirrhosis. The sixth, seventh, and eight cases in Frankfurt all involved having other health problems in seeking medical care. Nancy was selected as the sixth case. Nancy sought help due to lung and breathing problems, and was similar to the other women because she had children and was in a partnership at the time of the interview. Similar to Rachel, Nancy came from an African country and this provided a comparison of two women with some similarities in their life histories. Both Nancy and Rachel had their children after their HIV diagnosis and were members of Helping Hand. Nancy discussed issues of her HIV in relation to her migration experience to Germany of being fearful to disclose because of her uncertainty of the immigration law requirements for her to secure a permanent stay in Germany. Her migration experience was distinct from Rachel and she did not discuss coming to Germany as an asylum seeker. Nancy worked as a babysitter to send money back home to her family and appeared to have more freedom in her initial stay in Germany as compared to Rachel. Nancy and Rachel both described having serious health problems, which prompted their seeking medical care and appeared to facilitate their acceptance of treatment.

Nancy discussed her shock at diagnosis and provided social context. Nina had lived in Germany since the late 1990s and since then gotten married and started working. Then she began having constant chest problems, difficulties breathing, and occasional headaches. Nancy went to see a physician and the physician referred her to a lung specialist and the specialist told her she had to do some tests. After her tests, she was told she had to come to the clinic where she discovered that she was HIV-positive. Nancy described how the physician called her, and that it was difficult for the physician to tell her she had HIV. When she was diagnosed she felt shocked, she couldn't even cry because she did not even know how to take it.

The physician gave Nancy hope and told her that he could send her somewhere to get medication and that HIV did not mean her life was going to end. The physician told Nina this because she asked him how long she had to live and the physician told her she shouldn't worry about that, that there was medication in Germany, and that he would send her somewhere she could register so that she could receive help. It took Nancy time to do this [Sequential Report 6, p. 1]. Similar to Sarah, she did not tell anyone she had HIV. Nancy did not even tell her husband and reported that she had to think about "What to do immediately and because I was working it took me some weeks, six weeks because everything was too much for me" [Sequential Report 6, p. 1].

Information about medical treatment upon diagnosis served to redefine HIV from a death sentence to a chronic illness. Information exchange with physicians and other patients emerged as key to positive coping with HIV. HIV diagnosis was the starting point for participants where they drew on the social context, emotional context, and situational context of their diagnosis. The seventh case was that of George and his case was selected because he was a gay man living with HIV for a long period of time and also accepted his HIV. George's vivid descriptions of inhumane treatment when he was first treated in a German hospital and misdiagnosed with cancer introduced elements of histories of medical treatment in contextualizing current HIV treatment. George described having near death experiences in a descriptive way that added new dimensions to the analysis. George was brought to the emergency room and was close to death.

George recalled how he had sex one day with a man who was not his partner and two days later he was lying in bed with a 40 degree (Celsius) fever. George was hospitalized after his mother found him with a high fever at his home and called the ambulance. George was taken to a hospital where he described his treatment as inhumane.

Upon his arrival in the hospital, George recalled having eight to nine different physicians within a week and felt that the physicians did not treat him as a person. George was relocated to numerous floors of the hospital because no one could identify the cause of his sickness. They lost all of his paperwork and this was stressful for George to experience. George lost his white blood cells after three days and his hemoglobin was "not working" so the physicians thought he had cancer [Sequential Report 7, p. 2]. No one knew what was happening and George came to the emergency room. George felt close to death but he felt would have been able to accept death because it was not the first time he was close to death and he was used to this feeling.

Although there were rooms in the hospital, when the physicians thought that George may have had cancer they had George outside of a room, on the floor, as they took out his bone marrow in a very public and humiliating manner. George discussed the circumstances of being close to death and experiencing what he felt was inhumane and poor treatment when rendering his experience of being diagnosed with HIV. Although he defined HIV as unexpected, George expressed a sense of relief in being able to know the true cause of his sickness after experiencing such negative treatment in the hospital. Therefore, the immediate social context of poor medical treatment and an ambiguous cause of illness were conditions that shaped his response to his HIV diagnosis.

After five days of receiving different diagnoses and poor medical care, George was diagnosed with HIV. George reported that he was not too shocked because sex had been important in his life and he came from the 1980s and had heard about gay men and HIV so he was not surprised. George was sleeping with different people so he knew HIV could happen. George would get tested every six months and the results were negative. George couldn't identify exactly how he contracted HIV because he claimed to have practiced safe sex and to use condoms. This remained an unresolved issue for George, he knew who he contracted HIV from, but was unable to identify how he contracted HIV from this man. George described having the question of "Why me?" upon learning of his HIV. This was similar to Walter who had difficulties identifying a clear cause of his HIV infection. George's health status at the time of his diagnosis was greatly diminished and he lost a great deal of weight (twenty kilograms).

HIV diagnosis was a major turning point, often throwing participants into a new identity as someone with HIV. Overcoming a misalignment of identity was a major process involved in the negotiation of HIV. As discussed in the introduction chapter, misalignment of identity has been identified as part of transformational processes of identity, which involves feelings of shock, tension, shame, and self-questioning (Strauss 1997). The existential crisis to sense of self and to mortality was framed in the social context and personal histories of the participants, suggesting that in order to understand coping with HIV, individual and social biographies need to be examined.

Accordingly, HIV diagnosis was described as a catalyst for extreme emotional pain. David described an intense suffering upon learning about his HIV-positive status. For example, David discussed staying with a close friend for a week after his diagnosis and having severe emotional pain. David learned to keep the pain inside. To cry inside. "You learn to cry inside of you, you learn to keep the pain inside of you" [Substantive Report 8, p. 2]. David learned to deal with this emotional pain and felt it would be a lie if he would have said everything was ok when he was diagnosed with HIV because it was not easy. Therefore, emotions of shock and feeling overwhelmed were reported as being key to initial experience with HIV and these emotions tended to inhibit proactive behavior, even if temporarily, due to shock, denial, and emotional overload. Receiving information about HIV and having access to HIV medication helped participants to redefine HIV from a death sentence to a chronic illness.

Similar to Rachel and Nancy, David also had migrated from an African country but had migrated at a younger age and did not have HIV upon his arrival in Germany. Similar to Arthur and Sarah, David was educated and explained that he had a high-income and had a professional demeanor. David was a gay man but unlike the other gay men, he was not a white European man, he was black and of African descent. Similar to Walter, David had a distinctly active communicative scheme in his interview. Interestingly, David was an activist who had engaged in community work to raise awareness of HIV. However, unlike Walter, David accepted his HIV. David presented a unique case because of his discussion of the American and German health care systems, his activism, and the nonconsensual disclosure of his HIV status due to media coverage in a local newspaper. David discussed having a friend who traveled between the US and Germany who was a musician and received care at the clinic and it is likely that he was referring to Walter. David reported having health problems that motivated him to come to the hospital. When David was diagnosed, he was seeking care for pain in his legs that prevented him from walking. Health status appeared to play an important role in the decision to seek medical treatment, which then lead to HIV testing. Prior experiences in other treatment facilities that were not specialized in HIV were described as problematic. The Frankfurt participants framed their care at the HIV clinic in a positive light and described their medical care as a source of information, support, and care. There appeared to be greater continuity of care among the patients in Frankfurt who unlike the Miami sample did not discuss issues of having to change doctors because of their medical insurance coverage or financial barriers to treatment. This suggests that medical coverage affected continuity of care in this sample. The importance of social policy in affecting illness experience and medical treatment is discussed in more detail in the section on structural and material conditions of policy. In addition, mode of HIV transmission was a condition that affected how HIV diagnosis was experienced, contextualizing the meaning of HIV.

3.3.3   *Mode of HIV Transmission as Providing Context for HIV*

3.3.3.1   Voluntary versus Involuntary Sex

The mode of HIV transmission emerged as an important factor in participants' coping with HIV and the social context and meaning of their HIV diagnosis. Mode of HIV transmission was a condition that shaped biographical coping responses to HIV diagnosis. One set of conditions in mode of transmission was the distinction between voluntary and involuntary sexual contact. Walter, Chris, Arthur, George, and David all reported voluntary sexual behavior as the reason for their HIV. Chris, unlike Walter, accepted the reality of his HIV and explained that he caught HIV by engaging in a threesome. Unlike Walter, the gay men reported accepting their sexual lifestyle as a cause of their HIV transmission. Arthur described how he was "playing with fire" and living a life of "sex, drugs, and rock and roll":

> "I've got a couple of friends of course who are HIV-positive (-) also HIV-negative guys (-) I've been open to most of them as well (---) certain (-) certain situations you can't control what's going on and uh sex and drugs and rock and roll (-) things happen (-) shit happens as well infection wise." [Transcript 4; lines 94-98]

Arthur elaborated:

"Well scared in the way of I was forty (-) wait I was exactly forty when I got the diagnosis and I knew that I was playing with fire if you call it that way. (-) uh so in a way I was kind of expecting it to happen someday but not so early (-) and uh I had worked my whole life since I was about fifteen and uh that shouldn't have been it at all that should have been something else (-) and I thought 'Ok probably two or three or four or five years more then I've had it' I still had to work." [Transcript 4; lines 124-128]

Arthur felt that he was living a risky life. He was almost expecting to get HIV because he was "playing with fire" and yet he did not expect to get HIV "so early." HIV was something that he anticipated could "happen" in an ambiguous future time. Therefore, HIV appeared to be conceptualized as an external event due to "bad luck" that happened to Arthur. Understanding the cause of HIV infection appeared to play an important role in participants' contextualization of HIV into their biographies and coping responses.

Arthur took care in the introduction of his narrative to explain that he had been gay his whole life, so why did he feel that getting HIV at the age of forty was so early in his life? It is possible that he claimed to have expected for HIV to "happen" but at the time was in denial of the reality that HIV could be a consequence of his risky behavior. Similar to the manner in which a cigarette smoker may know that smoking could lead to cancer and yet continues to smoke despite this risk due to the chance that they can still engage in the behavior they desire without any consequences, Arthur may have continued to play with fire. By having an awareness of the risk of HIV and yet at the same time pushing HIV away into an indefinite future, which he hoped or felt would never come to actualize itself in his life, Arthur was able to live a life of risk without an immediate fear of death. Chris also was aware that he was putting himself at risk via risky sexual contact:

"There's a difference I think (-) a lot of people might um (--) be like how do I say it? Some people get infected and they didn't even do anything like out of a hospital or an operation or whatever you know I feel sorry for those people (-) like um If my mom says 'Oh how did you get it?' 'Ok we had a threesome with someone' yes it was stupid maybe um so I got it and I can live with it (-) It's not like I tell myself 'Why did I get it? And I feel horrible and shouldn't have done it (-)' No like I'm absolutely ok with it (-) I just feel sorry for those people who really didn't do anything and got it by mistake and that they're getting treated like they're people in second class." [Transcript 3; lines 277-283]

Chris distinguished himself from those who have been infected with HIV due to an operation or other means that he felt are outside of that person's control. Chris admitted to having a threesome, accepted his illness, and acknowledged the role his behavior had in leading to his new life with HIV. However, for those who were infected in contexts beyond their control, he felt they must deal with more existential questions of why they must live HIV, whereas he could accept that he had HIV. Mode of HIV transmission can be a condition for contextualizing HIV into biography. When the mode of HIV transmission was identifiable and viewed as the result of one's own actions it appeared easier to accept than when the cause of HIV infection was ambiguous or due to circumstances out of one's control. Chris sympathized with those infected who were not responsible for their HIV status because he felt they did nothing to deserve HIV and yet were being treated as "second class."

Chris could cope with his HIV because he knew why he had HIV and accepted the reasons leading to his HIV infection. David also accepted the reasons for his HIV, unprotected sex with another man, and could cope with his HIV. Conversely, Walter denied the existence of his HIV as he debated heterosexual sex as a potential cause but moved away from this explanation. For example, Walter's doctor told Walter about a symptom of HIV where one becomes very ill for a week and then feels better. Experiencing this symptom lead Walter to debate if he had had an adverse reaction to a generic sleeping medication or if he had been infected with HIV by past sexual partner. Thus, the origins of Walter's HIV infection were ambiguous, sexual contact was debated as the cause of HIV infection but was pushed out of Walter's awareness.

George also had an idea of how he came into contact with HIV. George could identify the man who gave him HIV but was unable to identify how exactly he was infected due to his practice of safe sex. George felt the need to learn that "safe sex isn't safe sex, it's safer sex" (Sequential Report 7, p. 5). The ambiguous cause of HIV despite his own effort to prevent HIV transmission was a cause of a difficulty in George's contextualization of HIV infection into his own biography. George reported that the physicians never asked him how he got HIV but he would like to know. This bothered George, he explained that it was important to know because he did not want to do it again because he did not want to give someone else HIV. George felt that whatever he did was a mistake and so he needed to know how he was infected. George used condoms, there were no accidents that he knew of, and he could not answer this question of infection.

Overall, the men interviewed tended to emphasis voluntary sexual contact as a mode of transmission of HIV, whereas the women discussed involuntary sexual contact or minimized the importance of sexual contact as mode of transmission and focused instead on other aspects of their HIV experiences. In contrast to the men interviewed, Rachel and Sarah report that they contracted HIV via involuntary sexual contact. Rachel's experience was more violent and clearly involuntary as she was victim of sexual violence. Sarah was married but felt betrayed by her husband and so defined her HIV infection in a context of betrayal and deception on the part of her husband. Nancy did not discuss how she contracted HIV but was married at the time of her diagnosis living in Germany.

For Rachel, the cause of her HIV infection was painfully clear. This traumatic experience however provided a clear cause of HIV. There was no ambiguity surrounding Rachel's cause of HIV infection. Although this experience was clearly traumatic and Rachel was an unwilling participant in the context of her HIV infection the clear cause of her HIV infection provided an identifiable and comprehensible context for the cause of her HIV. Sarah described how her deceased husband infected her with HIV against her knowledge in the misleading safety of her marriage. Sarah viewed her HIV infection as a betrayal and attributed the cause her husband's HIV to his perceived infidelity and bi-sexuality.

The involuntary nature of both women's diagnoses involved elements of violation and betrayal, suggesting that women with HIV may have unique needs when diagnosed with HIV. However, additional analyses of women are needed and this cannot be generalized to other women as the cases selected were exceptional cases and selected for analysis on the basis of their exceptional nature and challenging existing conceptions of HIV. Mode of HIV transmission emerged as a condition which affected the context of disease, which in turn was related to how agency was realized and drawn upon to act upon the external world. Another dimension of the mode of HIV transmission was gay versus straight sexual contact and is discussed below.

3.3.3.2   Gay versus Straight Sexual Contact as Mode of HIV Transmission

Gay sex as a mode of HIV transmission appeared to be related to an acceptance of HIV and integration of HIV into biography and identity. Chris, Arthur, and David acknowledged the risky sexual behaviors they were engaged in and thus accepted their HIV. However, George could only identify the man who he contracted HIV from but not the mode of transmission because he claimed to engage in safe sex. For those who reported contracting HIV via heterosexual contact despite it being voluntary or involuntary in nature, described their HIV as not being as easily accepted initially. This may be due to the prevalence of stereotypes of HIV being an issue for the gay community. For straight people, having HIV presented an identity and group characteristic, being gay, which was not consistent with their conception of their self-view and was harder to process and accept. For instance, Sarah described her feeling that she was not a typical HIV case:

> "I've always been someone who uh is not very typical (-) or more atypical (slight laughter) being affected by HIV (-) so I've been treated very (-) very well really very kind and really friendly all the time (-) I think this is something that people still might think having HIV you (-) could be a drug addict or somehow having to do with homosexual scenes and it might be (-) I think it is even like that still." [Transcript 5; lines 499-503]

Sarah was aware of negative stereotypes of people with HIV and felt that she was a unique case which ran counter to these stereotypes. She was not a drug addict, she was not gay, she was a widowed woman with children who was infected by her deceased husband and felt that her life circumstances did not fit the stereotypes that were often applied to HIV. The social context of diagnosis played an important role in shaping participants' experiences with HIV. While gay sex as a mode of transmission appeared to facilitate acceptance of HIV, being gay was also described as an additional stressor that intersected with HIV. The negotiation of HIV and gay-related stigma is elaborated in the section on stigma. Sarah emphasized how because she broke HIV stereotypes and was not a typical case of someone with HIV.

Walter also discussed his management of his own self-view in relation to HIV-related stereotypes. Walter exhibited the possession of a lay theory of HIV patients as being dirty, irresponsible, and as being addicted to drugs. This view of people with HIV had serious implications for his view of himself as a clean, "normal" person. Indeed, he recounted his experience taking the train back from the doctor when he first learned he was HIV-positive:

> "You can't see anybody that has it, you don't know. I mean anybody can have it, anytime, anywhere, know what I'm saying you know when I found out that I supposedly had it, you know I was sitting on the train I was (-) I was you know on the train going home and I was looking like 'Maybe she got it' 'Maybe he got it' 'He could have it' 'She could have' know what I'm saying? You know these people could have it but just living life normal like (-) you know like that you know (-) it's just (-) it's it got me aware on that note. And then I'm like 'Anybody could have this' and I say 'Maybe they could conduct themselves the same way I'm conducting myself' with the awareness of me having this know what I mean? You never know. Cause there's nothing written on your head 'Yeah hello HIV, hello HIV' there's no marks on you." [Transcript 1; lines 806-823]

The above excerpt contains numerous conceptions of HIV. The ambiguity of HIV status was made clear, "anybody can have it, anytime, anywhere" there were no "marks" signifying a person's membership into the group of people living with HIV. Statuses that are ambiguous may be rendered as especially problematic especially in the case of HIV where the only existing conceptions of HIV are linked to de-legitimized and deviant statuses such as the image of the drug addict or gayness. Importantly, Walter discussed how his diagnosis made him "aware" of the ambiguity of HIV status group membership. Walter's existing conception of those with HIV was challenged and was no longer fully cohesive and became contested and problematized in his awareness. Thus, what was known about HIV became fundamentally challenged. Walter explained:

"So you can't look at a person. Some you may look at and be like 'Hmmm there's a possibility' 'You have something' you know what I mean? Like junkies and crackheads and you can look at that and tell, know what I mean? But a normal person [...] You would never know that you know? And because you do come in contact (-) you do come across (-) come in contact with it does not mean you're a junkie It doesn't mean that you're an addict or anything of this nature." [Transcript 1; lines 825-836]

Drug addicts were differentiated from those who are "normal." HIV group membership was ambiguous to Walter in terms of visibility but the image of the drug addict was a dominant factor distinguishing between those who were "normal" and those who could be held accountable for having contracted HIV. He elaborated:

"Who knows? Maybe you're out in the woods somewhere and cut something in some way and who knows? And it happened for me (-) it could just you know happen, know what I'm saying? It doesn't necessarily mean or have to be that you're a junkie or an addict or something like that. That I don't (-) it doesn't necessarily mean that, you know but I don't talk to nobody about it cause 'Why?' do (--) **they wouldn't understand me.**" [Transcript 1; lines 838-842]

Walter compared those who came across HIV in an accidental manner to drug addicts who could be held accountable for their HIV status. Walter considered himself as "normal" and because HIV entered his life, this brought him to the brink of an awareness shift in how he conceptualized people with HIV. HIV was now a condition that could potentially happen to anyone, it could be an accident, it happened to him so it could now happen to those who were "normal." Although Walter did not accept his HIV diagnosis as real and continuously acted to construct a reality where it was unreal, he was on the verge of a new group membership to the HIV community. His awareness of the possibility that this "virus" truly was within him challenged how he perceived people with HIV.

Walter's discussion of the imagery surrounding drug addiction and HIV also emphasized the marginalization and social distance towards those suffering from drug addiction.

The awareness of a new group membership may shape conceptions of PLWHA. Integrating new group conceptions may also play a role in how people come to terms with HIV and work to integrate this into their own personal biographies and identity. Indeed, self-view and presentation of self both emerged as important elements of HIV diagnosis and coping responses to HIV. A diagnosis of HIV involved an identification with a new social world and identity role of being someone who is HIV-positive. Existing conceptions of the self at diagnosis needed to be reconciled with new role definitions as participants adjusted to their new lives with HIV.

3.4   HIV as Existential Identity Threat

The process of negotiating identity emerged as an integral aspect of coming to terms with HIV diagnosis and was an enduring dilemma for participants. Because this process began upon the discovery of one's HIV status, the process of coming to terms with HIV as an existential identity threat is discussed here. When chronic illness is experienced as overwhelming and out of control it can correspond to a threat to self-conceptions and a reframing of illness experience (Charmaz 1991). This overwhelming trajectory of suffering can diminish feelings of autonomy and independence and damage reciprocity in social interaction, which can lead to additional strain (Freund and McGuire 1991). Presentation of self and threat to identity conceptions in description of diagnosis emerged as an important component of participant's' experiences. HIV was presented as an existential dilemma that extended beyond issues of mortality and death. HIV deeply affected participants' self-images and was related to the more general biographical processes of both a trajectory of suffering and of action. For example, Walter took care to present himself in a positive light before moving to a potential reason for his HIV-positive status:

> "How did I come in touch with this? I have no idea (-) I'm usually pretty persistent at what I do and how I do it even as far as staying away or (--) yeah just staying away from dirty things things that are not clean (-) so if I use public toilet If I had to sit down and defecate then I would use ah put paper on the toilet seat (-) you know things of this nature (-) I wouldn't just sit down (-) um you know I'm I'm pretty persistent (-) I was pretty persistent and protecting myself at least I thought I was (-) um the only way I could think of me having this was from sexual contact cause

I was (-) there's been times when I played with (--) (--) I took the risk and didn't use a condom and probably this is why this has happened (-) if this is really here." [Transcript 1; lines 15-24]

Walter debated how he might have possibly become infected if – as he emphasized – he actually was infected. He described his hygiene and cleanliness and presented himself as a "clean" and "persistent" person. He was conflicted in regards to how HIV became a part of his life and, as he described how he acted and what kind of person he was, built up an argument of how it would not be like him to have become infected. He discounted the credibility of his infection by presenting himself as a clean person, as a persistent and cautious person who stayed away from things that were dirty.

However, at the end of this statement he provided a potential cause of his HIV infection, sexual contact. There was an underlying paradox where Walter had a self-image of himself as clean and persistent and yet had to account for how he had come into contact with HIV. Walter attempted to present himself in a socially acceptable manner, as a cautious, legitimate person who did not deserve to have HIV. Walter did not begin with his narrative with sexual contact but instead started by defining himself in a positive light. Other participants struggled with misalignment of their identity and the new reality of HIV. The confrontation of a new identity as an HIV-positive person presented an existential identity threat where past conceptions of the self needed to be reconciled with conceptions of HIV. Conceptions of people with HIV among participants involved the images of homosexuality, sin, drug addiction, marginalization, being "dirty", and sexual irresponsibility.

Therefore, the process of negotiating this identity struggle closely relates to modified labeling theory, which argues that members of stigmatized groups hold the same conceptions as the public of the group to which they are becoming members, and that confronting these negative stereotypes is stressful and has serious consequences for self-view (Link et al. 1989). Furthermore, socialization is argued to lead to expectations of how those labeled with stigmatized social statuses believe they will be treated once they are labeled (Lemert, 1974; Link et al. 1989). Because biographical work involves integrating new conceptions of the self into personal biographies, biographical analysis explicates the processes involved in coping with new group membership as a person with a stigmatized status by emphasizing the importance of identity in coping.

HIV was described as a label that participants had control over because HIV was described as being ambiguous to identify. Participants explained that there were no "marks" or "signs" signaling to others that someone has HIV. For example, George did not want a "sign on his face" announcing to others that he had HIV and did not want HIV to become a part of how others defined him due to his anticipation of stigma. Anticipation of stigma can be rooted in expectations of how others react to HIV due to their negative conceptions of HIV. HIV was a status that participants selectively disclosed to an inner circle of trusted others in a context of safety. The identity as an HIV-positive person was carefully negotiated.

HIV infection can present an inherent paradox through the infliction of processes of suffering and potential threat to one's life, on the one hand, and one's own action that has brought about this prolonged state of a potential trajectory of suffering when the mode of HIV transmission is voluntary sexual contact. For instance, Walter was caught in limbo and unable to accept the reality of his HIV, which contributed to his maintenance of a construction of his HIV as an experiment. This process of identity struggle and group affiliation is discussed below.

The narratives prompted an investigation into the processes involved in identity formation and change as discussed by Strauss (1997). As Strauss (1997) posited, the development of identity can be conceived of as a transformation of identity. The new-found status as an HIV-positive person placed participants in a state of internal struggle or "misalignment" with their prior conceptions of self (Strauss 1997, p. 95). "Misalignment" was defined by Strauss as: "surprise, shock, chagrin, tension, bafflement, self-questioning." The diagnosis of HIV therefore represented what Strauss termed "challenges" that were involved in transformations of identity. This challenge was clear in the case of Walter whose conception of self was counter to his views of people with HIV. HIV status can serve as a private challenge with deep meaning, threatening former views of the world and of self.

Identity struggle upon HIV diagnosis was reported by participants. HIV was reported as shocking and throwing participants into a new, unknown social world – the world of HIV. The integration of past and present self was crucial to regaining a sense of coherence and stability in the face of existential crisis. The integration of a new identity as being HIV-positive was an essential part of biographical work. Integration of conceptions of self with one's conceptions of the social world of HIV was a struggle. In working out these difficulties in aligning a new, problematized group identity with their self-image participants: drew on their past and current conceptions of people with HIV (before and after diagnosis), their perceptions of how the public views people with HIV, and compared HIV to other chronic illnesses, as they worked to make sense out of what HIV meant for who they were and how others perceived them. Identity struggles were also rooted in time as time since diagnosis, generational cohort (diagnosed before versus after the advent of HAART), and age all played roles in adjustment to their lives with HIV. Coping with HIV is a major sociological issue because it involves processes of group identification, navigation between social worlds, and complex processes involving identity and agency, all of which are embedded in the personal and cultural historical context of HIV.

Identity struggles with new self-identification with the HIV-positive community were resolved in some cases. Importantly, the processes and conditions leading to the resolution of identity struggle varied among the cases analyzed, which emphasized the importance of personal biography in coping. This supports Corbin and Strauss' (1988) formulation of biographical work processes as distinct but overlapping, particularly emphasizing the processes of:

> "*Coming to terms* (arriving at some degree of understanding and acceptance of the biological consequences of actual or potential failed performances)" and "*reconstituting identity* (reintegrating identity into a new conceptualization of wholeness around the limitations in performance)." (p. 68 f.)

Acceptance versus denial of HIV status can be conceptualized as a result of how people negotiate the "coming to terms" and "reconstituting identity" biographical work processes. Walter's case was a clear example of denial. Walter emphasized the action scheme of his experience and how this perception of himself as an active person who took care of his life was central to his self-perception. Including his awareness of "being infected" into his self-perception, as a state of suffering and insecurity inflicted on him, was difficult for him. This might be one aspect of shutting the knowledge of his infection out of his full awareness context (Glaser and Strauss 1965) and making it seem unreal instead.

HIV presented a threat to self-concept involving a dangerous encounter with a new identity charged with threat to self-conception. Threat and danger was thus encountered both on the internal and relational-interactional level. As demonstrated in the case of Walter, there can be a constant danger in social interaction and in the perception and relation to self-concept. The strain in negotiating threat and danger to relations to self, self-conception, and to others can contribute to the construction of elaborate defenses affecting the action taken to cope with threat. Walter's collective identity as an African American man and musician presented with HIV highlighted this struggle. HIV can be a "stereotype threat" which involves the risk of confirming the possession of a negative group characteristic (Steele and Aronson 1995). For example, Walter presented himself as having a strong masculine, sexual, and responsible character and HIV was charged with images of homosexuality, drug addiction, and dirtiness.

Walter could not articulate why, but deep within in him was the undeniable feeling that he was betrayed, which was involved in his formation of HIV as an experiment. Interestingly, he relied on this feeling that existed within him to argue for the validity of the experiment construction. He described the clinic, there were students there, and it was a large medical facility. He could not say where this feeling that he was in an experiment came from. The feeling was "just within" him. Walter was partially in the "world of phantasy" as described by Schütz (1962), where his feeling was something that could not be contradicted because this feeling remained in a world of origin undefined and simply existed, thus evading contradiction (Schütz 1962, p. 237).

The construction of the experiment allowed Walter to reconcile his identity as a cautious, clean, and active person forced to contend with a circumstance that he felt he was placed in his against his will. This allowed him to maintain a strong self-image of himself as autonomous and strong. Paradoxically, by maintaining his identity as autonomous and strong, he refused to trust physicians and was ambivalent about his medical care. Walter did not admit any state of helplessness or need for care. Conversely, Rachel accepted her illness and felt that her physicians were some of the only people that she could trust besides her family. Rachel trusted the doctors out of her need for medical treatment and felt that without medical care she could not live. Therefore, Rachel's trust in physicians appeared to emerge from an instrumental need for care. Interestingly, Rachel framed her diagnosis as a relief and as a necessity to her survival as opposed to having an emphasis on feeling shocked and emotionally upset. These divergent reactions can be conceived of as processes rooted in the biographical structure of their life histories and experiences. For Rachel, the context of diagnosis was shaped by her need for medical care, her closeness to death, and the political violence in her native country, which lead to her encounter with HIV. In contrast, the processes of emotional shock and aversion to HIV diagnosis for Walter and Chris occurred in a context of good health, location in an industrialized nation with affordable and extensive health care services, and their sexual histories. Rachel had engaged in biographical work in order to "come to terms" with HIV because she accepted her HIV, understood her illness, and had worked to reconstitute her identity into a new cohesive conceptualization where she accepted the challenges HIV introduced into her biography.

Participants discussed difficulties in trusting others with their secret identity of HIV. In order to handle feelings of distrust, and to prevent the possibility of betrayal and exposed HIV status, they employed different strategies and these strategies shaped their social worlds and experiences. Walter described how he used what he called "ethical persuasion" a term he defined as his means of negotiating his secret of HIV by influencing social interactions so as to avoid the topic of HIV (Transcript 1, line 488). Rachel disclosed in a safe environment and accepted her membership in the HIV-positive community, which allowed her to transverse between these two social worlds.

Unlike Rachel, Walter did not fully accept his HIV status and did not identify himself as a member of the HIV-positive community. Walter's discussion of how "you can't see anybody that has it, you don't know" suggested that he was on the verge of awareness of his new life with HIV. Walter elaborated on his feelings of not having HIV and yet his diagnosis made him aware that anyone with a "normal" life could have HIV. Walter entered an unsafe world where his perceptions of the world as he knew it were deeply shaken as he lost his criteria for defining and categorizing people. His standards and distinctions of groups suddenly became unstable and he couldn't trust what was already known. His view of the world and his sense of belonging were in a state of confusion. Walter was avoiding the realization of being in a trajectory of suffering and was acting against his own benefit, instead of towards influencing the trajectory of suffering that he forced out of his awareness in order to keep a trajectory of suffering at bay. Walter was engaged in action in pushing HIV out of his awareness but he also was experiencing a loss of control and meaning. This tension between his argumentative activities and his action are discussed in more detail on the section on the reversal of agency.

Walter recounted his experience taking the train back from the doctor when he first learned he was HIV-positive. The ambiguity of HIV status was made clear, "anybody can have it, anytime, anywhere" there were no "marks" signifying a person's membership into the group of people living with HIV. Importantly, he discussed how his diagnosis made him "aware" of the ambiguity of HIV status group membership and yet he pushed this awareness away by adding "when I found out that I supposedly had it." Walter's perceptions of people with HIV became questionable. However, his conceptions of those with HIV were not fully cohesive and still remained somewhat contradictory.

Walter explained that in some cases it was possible to label someone as HIV-positive and he repeated his conceptualization of the drug addict as HIV-positive. Drug addicts were differentiated from those that were "normal." HIV-positive group membership was ambiguous to Walter in terms of visibility but the image of the drug addict was a dominant factor distinguishing between those who were "normal" and those who could be held accountable for having contracted HIV. Walter made a group distinction between normal people who come across HIV in an accidental manner and drug addicts who he held accountable for their HIV status. Walter considered himself as "normal" and because HIV entered his life, this brought an awareness shift in how he conceptualized people with HIV. HIV was on the verge of re-definition as a condition that could happen to anyone, it happened to Walter and so it could happen to those who were "normal." However, Walter remained ambivalent in his conception of HIV. Walter maintained a distinction between himself and the other patients he saw at the clinic:

"My personal, deep down inside, my instinct could be wrong but you know instincts usually don't lie. You know? Um I just feel I'm an experiment for some reason. I (-) I (-) I don't feel (-) I mean I see that are (-) that's in here when I come here to pick up this medication you know I come to speak to the doctor, I see the (-) I see the people and the people I see you can see you can 'wow ok' you can probably understand that you can probably (-) not that you can see a person as HIV because you really can't see it but you can kinda (-) you can look and 'ok' you can kinda see or kinda understand 'ok yeah maybe that could be' I am in a different class than people I've seen you know, I (-) I (-) I not saying that I'm better or below (-) I'm not saying none of that. I'm just (-) I'm just (-) I'm just another class, you know from the people that I see and I'm (-) I really, I really, I really can't grasp the fact that I have this, I really can't grasp this fact." [Transcript 1, lines 165-182]

He struggled and resisted being identified as having HIV as he shifted directly into his view of the patients at the clinic. Walter explicitly stated his difficulty grasping the reality of HIV. Walter resisted against identifying with the other patients. He was quick to correct himself and said he was not saying there was a hierarchical difference between him and the other patients but still maintained a distinction from them. Both Walter and Chris used the term "class" when describing distinctions made in determining HIV group membership. Chris stated "I just feel sorry for those people who really didn't do anything and got it by mistake and that they're getting treated like they're people in second class." Accountability for HIV appeared to be a factor in evaluating people with HIV. Chris sympathized with those who he felt were not accountable for their HIV and yet were judged and treated as "second class" whereas Walter maintained that he was not superior but in a "different class" than the other patients. Both Chris and Walter also made distinctions between themselves and others with HIV. Chris saw himself as responsible for his HIV status and accepted it but did not feel he was treated as "second class" and Walter maintained distance from group membership by claiming to be in a "different class."

Conceptions of HIV and their relationship to identity can be viewed as a part of an ongoing process of group identification. Identity and group identification appeared to share an ongoing relationship and this dynamic process was important in reconstituting identity into a coherent sense of belonging based on intersectional biographical position. Faced with a new social world, new group, and new self, participants related their views of their selves to their conceptions of HIV. Identity and group identification appeared to have a dynamic relationship, shaping each other in an ongoing process over time. This process may unfold with an initial feeling of being dissimilar to people with HIV and then moving to an awareness of the possibility of similarity between the group and the self, and then moving to the issue of dealing with the implications of what it means to now be similar to the new group of HIV-positive people for identity.

The internal, instinctual part of the self or as Mead (1934) conceptualized it the "I" was related to a new generalized other and the "Me" or social self also shifted and it was necessary to adjust strategies in negotiating reality to help the "I" to settle into the new identity as an HIV-positive person. Therefore, individual and collective identity may be conceptualized as interrelated concepts and as process based concepts which share an ongoing, dynamic relationship. Positive group identification with HIV was related to resolving identity struggle and these conflicts in group identification required reconciliation. On the structural and historical levels, the meaning of group membership was rooted in social conceptions and political movements rooted in power struggles to legitimatize respective social worlds such as HIV and homosexuality, highlighting the role of social arenas in social reality as formulated by Strauss (1993).

Participants discussed how HIV support groups were important in facilitating coping and acceptance of HIV. Rachel, David, and Nancy described how the social support intervention Helping Hand helped them to accept their new lives with HIV and to feel more comfortable seeking HIV-related treatment and services. Helping Hand provided a new discourse that affected identity and group identification, and which emphasized the importance of discourse and raised awareness on the immediate chances patients perceived and their coping abilities. More precisely, Helping Hand opened a new social world to participants where they could discuss their HIV in a context characterized by mutual acceptance and understanding. Helping Hand provided patients with a safe place where they could exchange experiences, ideas, and information thus providing members with a new discourse about HIV.

Through developing a sense of belonging, members learned to relate in more positive ways to others with HIV and to more easily integrate HIV into their own self-concept. By developing an understanding that they were not alone in their life situation, and by exchanging information and gaining access to this new source of social capital, members' awareness of their opportunities and potential to cope with HIV were enhanced. As Sacks (1967) suggested, having someone to turn to for support was discussed as helpful. For example, by actively seeking help when feeling they had no one to turn to, Helping Hand provided someone turn to for support. Participating in Helping Hand helped participants to become aware that HIV was a condition that could be negotiated and was not a death sentence or the end of their hopes for a normal life. The resolution of identity struggle and processes in self-discovery and acceptance emerged as key to biographical action process structures and involved biographical work.

Participation in support groups like Helping Hand can help to alleviate the strain of maintaining the secret of HIV in daily life. Separating different spheres of life and social identities was reported as stressful and producing an additional between social worlds and senses of belonging. Separation strain can be seen as on a continuum and participants needed a way to negotiate this strain. Helping Hand provided a "safe place" to reveal the secret of HIV, thus alleviating the strain of maintaining a secret life of HIV. Indeed, Riemann and Schütze (1991) argued that a trajectory of suffering involves feelings of separation which occur alongside becoming strange to oneself and exploring a new and strange world. Riemann and Schütze (1991) also argued that enduring feelings of self-alienation can create strain, facilitating changes in the definition of personal identity.

In contrast to the members of Helping Hand, Walter put all his energy in maintaining this secret and did not have a safe place to disclose his HIV status. The constant maintenance of the secret of HIV contributed to his paranoia and deep distrust of others and his own alienation. However, Walter's distrust of medicine was rooted in a kernel of truth, the historical racism in the U.S. and abuse of African Americans in unethical research projects. Although rooted in a truth, this distrust prevented Walter from taking action to regain control over his life.

The negotiation of strained identity relations or of reintegrating and recasting of biography was deeply rooted in correcting misalignment of identity. This emerged as a major theme in development of a transition out of a trajectory of suffering and into regaining control over participants' lives. Also, because this strain was present on biographical, social-contextual, and relational levels biographical process structures of action also developed on these levels as this strain was overcome. In addition, identity theorists have emphasized the close link between identity and action, the resolution of identity crisis can be central to understanding how empowerment is created by social actors and helps them to work to escape from trajectories of suffering thus enhancing their life conditions (Hogg et al. 1995; Stryker 1980). Overcoming misalignment of identity can help people with HIV to escape a trajectory of suffering and to gain a sense of control over their lives. Because identity and action have been discussed as having a deep relationship, developing a meaningful sense of belonging can help PLWHA to engage in proactive behavior to improve their life circumstances, such as involvement in support groups, adherence to treatment, and other healthy behaviors. Specifically, by accepting themselves and having an understanding of their needs and the actions needed to achieve their goals, participants were better able to exit a trajectory of suffering and to take action geared at improving their life conditions.

Because HIV often involved painful and difficult biographical experiences, participants often faded their HIV out of their awareness contexts (Glaser and Strauss 1965). Applying the analytical concepts of a conditional matrix and of process structures of biographical experience enabled an analysis of the life conditions and biographical processes that were related to participants regaining a sense of control over their lives. Following the guidance of Schütze (2007), an analysis of pragmatic refraction allowed for an in-depth analysis beyond a description of participants' experiences. I related the descriptive level of interviewee's experiences with their context of life experience and the overall biographical structure of their interviews to generate theoretical insights into their biographical experiences.

3.5   Part 2: Biographical Process Structures

The analytical concepts of biographical processes facilitated an analysis of how people experienced their HIV and for the identification of processes that were involved in biographical adjustment to illness, which was an ongoing process. Participants had to take continuous action to maintain their action and to avoid falling into a trajectory of suffering. HIV was not a status that was static but rather it was an ongoing aspect of people's lives. The analytical concept of various process structures allowed for an examination of what conditions were supportive for interviewees. As discussed in the methodology chapter, process structures are distinct but can be overlapping. Drawing on the biographical approach, there are four process structures: action process structures, trajectories of suffering, institutional expectation patterns, and creative metamorphosis of identity (Schütze 2007).

Biographical process structures are especially useful in identifying what can be supportive to people facing challenges in their lives. Action process structures involve taking action to purposely shape one's life circumstances and trajectories of suffering involve a loss of control and meaning over one's life. By examining such processes we can better understand what resources and conditions are supportive in enhancing feelings of autonomy and personal transformative potential. Also, as will be discussed later in this comparison, creative metamorphosis of identity emerged and involved a deep exploration of the inner self and its capabilities. Other transformative biographical processes such as creative production and spiritual journeys were emphasized. These two process structures (action and transformative) emerged as important to participants' lives with HIV. However, institutional expectation patterns where one follows a sequence of institutionalized roles such as student to apprentice to worker were not emphasized in by participants. The following chapters discuss the process structures which emerged in participants' narratives.

Biographical work and its close tie to action were characterized by biographical process structures identified in the cases analyzed. Biographical work such as contextualizing, coming to terms, reconstituting identity, and recasting biography as described by Corbin and Strauss (1988) were related to biographical process structures of action schemes and to transformative processes. The shift from a biographical process structure of trajectory of suffering to that of action emphasized the importance of the relationship between biographical work and process structures of action in this analysis. Similarly, Schütze (2007) posited that biographical work is indeed related to action schemes as he stated:

"Biographical work is basically an inner activity of mind and emotional psyche, and this inner activity is essentially constituted by conversation with significant others and oneself. In life situations of biographical crisis, biographical work can become the explicit and central action scheme of cognitively and emotionally ordering one's own life; in smoothly ongoing life situations it may be just a quick deliberation and recollection connected to the focus on other activities, or it may even be subliminal. The capacity as well as the incapacity of doing biographical work is very much conditioned by the course of the former life history and its involved learning processes as well as by the respective accidental and structural barriers for learning processes." (p. 7)

Schütze (1981; 1984) identified and developed biographical process structures as analytical concepts to facilitate the analysis of biographical experience, including different types of biographical action schemes. Furthermore, Schütze (2007) argued that biographical process structures were important principles which order life history. One biographical process structure was that of biographical action schemes where people seek to influence and actively take control over their lives. The biographical process structures of action identified in the analysis of the narratives were embedded in individual and social conditions, and these processes were portrayed through the use of cognitive figures in narration such as, social structures, frames of experiences, and the overall life history of interviewees (Schütze 1984).

Biographical work aimed at establishing coherence of biographical situation, identity and belonging, acceptance of HIV, and understanding how to maintain a fulfilling life despite HIV emerged in my analysis as an important aspect of action. The biographical process structures of action identified in the narratives can be conceptualized as processes which operated on the biographical, social-contextual, relational, and structural levels. Biographical process structures of action schemes were an important part of participants' experiences with HIV and the analysis of participants' narratives generated the conceptualization of different process structures of action. Importantly, there was a tension within trajectory of suffering processes, which allowed for the emergence of unforeseen transformations under certain conditions as participants attempted to regain control over their lives. The following chapters discuss action process structures and process structures related to transformative processes such as creative metamorphosis of identity, creative production, and spirituality. Also, the importance of material resources as supportive to action processes is discussed.

3.5.1   Biographical Action Process Structures

3.5.1.1   "Helping Hand" and Support Seeking

Helping Hand, an on-site program, was described as being beneficial to participants' coping with HIV and regaining a sense of control over their lives. Other forms of support seeking, such as seeking treatment and information from physicians facilitated acceptance of HIV, positive group identification with others living with HIV, and action. For example, Rachel's near-death experiences and hardships in her native country and upon her arrival in Germany, indicated a context of helplessness. Rachel's need for survival motivated her to take control over her life as manifested by her actions taken to seek medical support, leave her native country, come to Germany, maintain her medical treatment, and to engage in the Helping Hand support group. Seeking support helped Rachel to regain control over her life and to escape the trajectory of suffering inflicted upon her as a result of sexual violence and HIV transmission. Rachel described:

> "The thing which has helped me now is not very far it's not a long time (-) it's ah (blows nose) from before (-) last year when I came here to doctor and the doctor told me about this Helping Hand (-) yeah (-) this is the big thing which has to get me more ah so I feel better (-) when I'm here (-) I feel (-) I feel well (-) I feel good (-) and if I don't (-) go and tell the people I can see friends but I leave this point away." [Transcript 2, lines 157-164]

Based on my knowledge, the physicians at the clinic were instructed to refer patients with migration backgrounds to Helping Hand. When Rachel was at Helping Hand she felt "well" and "good." Although Rachel had friends outside of the hospital she did not tell them she had HIV. Rachel further elaborated on her reasons for not disclosing to people outside of the clinic her HIV status:

> "Yeah I even (other helping hand member) told me 'No you can tell the people and if you don't tell a person you cannot know how they will react' But I fear this reaction I don't know how the person can react to me because the (-) what I've experienced before is nothing good." [Transcript 2, lines 166-169]

Rachel had experienced significant weight loss, which identified and marked her by others as being sick and subsequently isolated her. Spatial alienation due to dispersal programs in Germany restricted her movement and structured her daily life in difficult, coercive ways, took away her privacy in medication taking, and placed her far from her only source of support.

Despite Rachel's helplessness and vulnerability, she managed to draw upon her inner strength, to shift her awareness to an awareness of her agency, and to take action to improve her life circumstances by seeking medical support and becoming an active member of the HIV-positive community. Taking action can be conceptualized as an enactment of agency. Thus, the term "enacted agency" was used because agency was conceptualized as process-based involving: first the awareness of agency developing and then a decision to "enact" or utilize agency in taking action to regain control over life circumstances.

Rachel could have chosen to not seek care and to not continue on, but her desire to live motivated her to take action by seeking medical support and later engaging in the Helping Hand support group. Furthermore, without the conditions of the possibility of immigration to Germany, access to quality medical care, and referral to the support group of Helping Hand, Rachel's potentiality for exerting change in her life would have been fundamentally limited. Rachel's effectiveness in shaping her life circumstances by seeking treatment, immigrating to a new country, learning a new language, and being active in her care may also have been due to a deep awareness and sensitivity of her needs. Unlike Walter, Rachel was attuned to her needs because she accepted her present self and circumstances instead of rebelling against her current identity. She accepted the reality of HIV and acted continuously to improve her life circumstances. Therefore, acceptance versus denial may be related to issues of misalignment between the past, present, and future self, affecting self-views and action.

David also felt that participating in Helping Hand was an important positive life change. When David was initially diagnosed he was emotionally devastated and was crying, crying all the time, he didn't want to cry but he couldn't keep it inside. The worst part for David was that he cried in a dream. He explained that he would wake up after having horrible dreams about HIV with pressure surrounding him. While dreaming, David would cry and the pillow would be wet with his tears as he would awaken. David felt that these dreams were one of the strangest experiences he had in his life and this is why he decided to change. Because during the day he was crying and even in his dreams he wept, and so it was time to change and to accept his HIV.

David began to attend Helping Hand meetings and felt that joining Helping Hand made him more confident. He no longer visited the clinic in shame and embarrassment with his head down. Instead, David talked to the other patients and gained support from learning about HIV from people who had HIV for decades. He also enjoyed giving support to newly diagnosed patients, which he reported doing the same day we interviewed. David reported talking with another man newly diagnosed and how talking to people about HIV was important to him. David talked to a man who just got HIV a few weeks ago at the time of the interview and they talked for an hour and this man also joined Helping Hand. David felt that joining Helping Hand made this man a whole new person.

Helping Hand was a major source of support for participants who were a part of the program. The clinic during the time of the interviews was busy, with numbers of patients coming in daily and physicians working long hours to provide treatment. Despite this overload of work, the physicians managed to provide quality medical care as reported by participants. Before Rachel participated in Helping Hand she was scared to seek medical care and services for her HIV she described:

> "Helping Hand helped me in the way that I can (--) yeah before I used to only come here to doctor (-) even the patients themselves (-) I didn't (-) I never used to talk to them and that I think is for many of us here (-) we see each other but we just go away (-) nobody wants to talk to the other you don't even know where the person comes from they yeah (-) but now I just talk to anybody (-) so I don't care because I know everybody whose here we are all the same (-) the person is either a doctor or a patient (-) before it was not like that." [Transcript 2, lines 353-364]

Participating in Helping Hand changed the way Rachel interacted and related with the other patients at the clinic and reduced her shame and fear of being seen seeking care. Prior to her involvement in Helping Hand, Rachel defined people at the clinic only as doctors or patients. However, after she joined Helping Hand Rachel interacted with the other patients in a more intimate way and this opened new possibilities for her relationships and increased her identification with other people living with HIV. Rachel redefined her group conceptions from the simple dichotomy of patients versus doctors at the clinic, to patients as people with whom she discussed her problems and fears with. Rachel identified with the HIV-positive community and could socialize and feel free to be open about her HIV status. Accordingly, safe, supportive groups may open new communities and worlds of possibilities to those who otherwise may live in isolation or have no safe place to discuss their lives with HIV. Entering Helping Hand helped to redefine the way Rachel identified with the other patients and gave her access to membership in the HIV-positive community in a safe place where everyone was the same and she did not have to fear being identified as being different or being excluded.

By being social and interactive within the HIV-positive community, Rachel took control over her life by extending her social networks and mastery over HIV. This indicated a dialectic that emerged in comparing the cases of Rachel and Walter. Rachel accepted that she was in need of help and receiving this help then increased her possibilities of social contact by widening the sphere of social interaction available for her to be active in. In contrast, because Walter resisted care, he was acting against his own intention, for control over his life and was restricted on what he could say to whom and on an existential level on the kind of person he was. This was because Walter felt he was living a lie so partly knew he was no longer who he used to be and yet was not able to accept that he could be in a position of need, and in turn this decreased his possibilities of taking action by utilizing the resources available in the HIV-positive community. Rachel elaborated:

"And even now um after I researched everything I ah can go to (--) we have ah how do they call it? AIDS Help something like that yeah (-) they (-) in every (-) in every city they have that an office for ah for people who have AIDS but before I could not enter that office though they can do many things (-) they help (-) they counsel the people if you have problems (-) or even for us that don't know the language they can read for you the letters, translate it (-) but for me it was hard (-) I used to think if I enter this ah this door maybe somebody see me from behind and then go out and say 'Ah I saw (Rachel) going to AIDS help'." [Transcript 2, lines 366-378]

Before joining Helping hand, Rachel was scared that she would be seen receiving help from the AIDS Help office and that other people would identify her as having HIV. Her fear of being exposed as HIV-positive was so powerful that it prevented her from seeking support. The office provided translational services for people whose first language was not German. Rachel discussed earlier in her interview how language was important for her, and that she learned German primarily so that she could be more autonomous in her HIV treatment. Therefore, her fear of detection was so great that it prevented her from utilizing a service she could have benefited greatly from. Seeking support, identifying with other patients, and accepting HIV helped Rachel to overcome her fear of detection and stigma which were major barriers that prevented her from seeking help.

In contrast, George was not a member of Helping Hand and reported similar fears of being identified while seeking care. George did not want to be seen coming to the clinic and was fearful of being seen. David reported that he believed that for many people the fear of being seen using HIV services is a major issue. Group identification with the HIV-positive community and the reduction of fear of being seen using services were important in helping participants to ability to regain control over their treatment.

Rachel described how another Helping Hand member provided her with a reason to not be afraid of being seen going to AIDS Help by telling Rachel that if anyone were to tell others that they had seen Rachel at AIDS Help, then they themselves would be placing their own reputation at jeopardy. Membership in Helping Hand reduced Rachel's fear of being exposed as HIV-positive, which enhanced her use of AIDS services. Therefore, socially supportive groups can help to facilitate enhanced well-being by helping people to cope with their illness and also to feel more comfortable utilizing health care services. Support seeking can be part of a process of regaining control over illness trajectories. Being comfortable with HIV and reducing fear of stigma can further empower patients to become more active in their treatment. For example, I asked Rachel if Helping Hand took away her fear of having other people know about her HIV status and she responded:

"Though I won't go to the person and say 'Yes I'm positive' but if I go there so I don't care whose going out to talk about me that is something that's different was not like before" [Transcript 2; lines 398-401].

Rachel still feared telling people about her HIV status but Helping Hand helped her to feel more comfortable when going to HIV services. Rachel no longer cared who may see her going to AIDS Help but still she would not openly tell her HIV status to others. I asked Rachel if Helping Hand had made her stronger and she agreed that it had. I probed and asked if Helping Hand had empowered her and Rachel replied:

" I used to never attend anything about it because sometimes I used to get letters here when they have uh a festival here (-) for the children and uh summer fest or something like that I never used to attend but now I just I know 'Yeah this is this day I want to go there' yeah (-) because I know when I go there I have fun with the people here and I have more fun here than as when I am with other people who are positive (-) who are negative." [Transcript 2, lines 407-418]

Rachel's group identification with the other patients enhanced Rachel's relationships with others with HIV and allowed her to have access to a new community. Rachel brought her children to these group activities and felt comfortable with and enjoyed socializing with the other members. Rachel even had "more fun" with members of Helping Hand than with HIV-negative people, which suggests that Rachel's ties to the HIV-positive community were positive and enhanced her well-being.

Nancy, another member of Helping Hand, reported that her participation in Helping Hand helped her to cope with HIV. Nancy said that Helping Hand helped her because she met people with similar problems and everyone talked about themselves in an open and comfortable setting where they could discuss almost everything about themselves. Nancy told the other members of the group about herself and about her medication. Some people talked about problems with their medication such as feeling dizzy. Everyone at the meetings would talk about themselves without being afraid and most people talked to people about HIV for the first time and they felt at home and accepted. Nina described how some people in the meetings would talk about how when they would tell their physicians they had HIV the physicians would push them out, that at least two people talked about this issue, which was similar to her own experience at the dentist where she was refused treatment due to her HIV status.

Because Nancy heard the stories from others with similar experiences, it made her feel like there were others who were in her situation, and gave her a group she could relate to. An important aspect of group membership in Helping Hand was the exchange of information. Nancy explained how they exchanged ideas about how to take care of problems they faced. For example, they discussed which doctors to disclose their HIV status to and those to whom they should not disclose. Members discussed their rights as patients. As long as their physician at the clinic knew, they did not have to tell other doctors about their HIV status and participants developed strategies to protect themselves from stigma. Nancy reported that members talked about topics that gave everyone strength and that many people left these lessons feeling more positive. From the meetings, Nancy met a few friends and they still talked and exchanged information at the time of the interview. This was important because some things Nancy could tell a physician "I feel like this, I feel like that" but maybe the physician wouldn't understand it "fast" because physicians likely themselves did not take the medicine (Sequential Report 6, p. 7). But if a person took the same medicine as Nancy did then she could exchange ideas with other patients about her care.

3.5.1.2   Group Identification and Social Support

Similar to the Frankfurt sample, Miami participants discussed issues of group identification and its relation to involvement in support groups. Sharing the social positions of HIV status and gender with others were not sufficient in creating an atmosphere of community and group solidarity that could help facilitate a socially supportive environment. Descriptions of others with HIV suggested that some participants internalized the negative stereotypes of people with HIV as being careless, irresponsible, dirty, uneducated, and addicted to drugs. Internalizing this negative imagery surrounding HIV and applying it to others appeared to be a barrier to relating to others with HIV. Such barriers are problematic because group identification was important in regards to involvement in support groups and acceptance of HIV.

Participants in Frankfurt also made distinctions between themselves and the other patients at the clinic and the more their self-concept differed from their conception of HIV and of the other patients, the more distant they were and the less involved they were with the other patients. Sociodemographic characteristics such as race/ethnicity, gender, and socioeconomic status can affect how comfortable people feel in specific support settings and processes of group identification. The fear of being seen using AIDS services was discussed in both the Frankfurt and Miami samples. Fear of stigma can be a barrier preventing participation in support groups and other health services. Utilization of support services was a powerful resource for people in both samples.

Support seeking and being actively involved in support groups was related to healthy and productive lifestyle changes and helped participants to maintain a positive outlook. The importance of a good fit between support group and personal preference was emphasized. In addition to issues of race and class similarity as being factors in relating to support groups, identifying with the method of support was reported as important. Being engaged in support groups appeared to have numerous benefits. Some benefits of being in a support group were being able to share experiences, being inspired by other's stories, relating to others, working on the self and emotions, and an increase in social networks.

3.5.1.3   Medicine as a Source of Support: The Need for Information in Treatment and Positive Views of Current Care

Participants discussed the importance of medical care as a source of support. Overall, participants discussed their current treatment at the clinic in Frankfurt in a positive light. For example, Chris explained that going to the clinic was "one of the best things" that happened to him. Similar to Rachel, Chris felt "really good here" he had "a really good feeling." David also reported a highly positive view of his care at the HIV clinic. Support, information, solutions, and understanding were key factors that shaped how participants responded to care. Chris desrcibed negative experiences with physicians in the past and compared them with his care at the clinic as he explained:

> "When I came here to the clinic to talk to the doctor like after I walked out of the room I was like 'Wow this really isn't a big deal' (-) it's like they have medication for it, they have treatment like they're being very supportive like they're open to all questions they will try to answer any question as good as they can and it gives you a secure feeling so (--) I think that's the main part like having a place you can go to um where people understand you (-) where people are supportive (-) they help you and they actually know what they're doing because when I got tested I just went to the ah regular doctor and they were like 'So what are you going to do?' and I was like 'Why are you asking me what I'm gonna do? Like you're the doctor you're supposed to have solutions or like ideas for me where to go'." [Transcript 3, lines 80-87]

When Chris obtained information from the doctors about HIV his conception of HIV changed, he began to feel that HIV was something that could be treated and lived with. The support that the doctors gave him was important and he felt that the doctors at the clinic here were supportive, understanding, and willing to answer his questions and this support and care gave him a "secure feeling." Support seeking and establishing relations of care with medical professionals were influential in helping Chris to come to terms with his HIV diagnosis. Chris felt that doctors should have solutions and provided care and felt that the physicians at the clinic who specialized in HIV provided him with better care than the "regular doctor." Specialist care was discussed as valuable to patients who felt that physicians who specialized in HIV and infectious diseases were more informed about HIV, not stigmatizing, and provided quality medical treatment and information about HIV, which helped participants to redefine their HIV from a death sentence to a chronic illness. This support and information helped participants to regain a sense of control over their lives and to make sense of their HIV.

David also emphasized the importance of having information about HIV upon diagnosis. Although David claimed to have knowledge of HIV prior to his diagnosis and to know on some level that HIV was not a death sentence, he was still fearful that he would die from HIV. David reported that obtaining information from members in Helping Hand greatly improved his coping with HIV. Nancy also discussed the importance of having information about HIV and sharing information with other patients. Therefore, information obtained from fellow patients and medical staff can help to enhance coping with HIV, which was reported as being critical upon initial diagnosis by participants. Receiving support from intimate partners, children, and medical staff was instrumental in helping participants to regain a sense of control over their lives and was related to biographical process structures of action.

For example, Nancy explained how another member of Helping Hand told the rest of the group that if they felt tired to take a type of tea in the morning for energy and how members exchanged many ideas. Nina felt she received a lot of help from them her fellow Helping Hand members. When Nancy told the group members she had twins they were surprised and she showed them pictures of her children. Nancy felt she had to show the other group members how someone with HIV could have HIV-negative twins who could survive. Nina emphasized that Helping Hand was "a good thing" (Substantive Report 6, p. 7). I asked if Helping Hand empowered her and Nancy responded that it had because she came to know that she was not alone, that there were other mothers who had HIV, and everyone talked about relationships and their partners and "everyone talked about their own life experience" [Substantive Report 6, p. 7].

Creating a collective meaning and a sense of belonging among patients was expressed in the discourse of Helping Hand where members related to each other's experiences, exchanged information, and developed strategies for overcoming challenges. Helping Hand provided a new discourse, which affected individual and collective identities, raising awareness of the immediate chances participants perceived and enhancing their ability to negotiate their HIV. Because individual identity and collective identity shared a dynamic relationship, shaping each other in a process-based manner over time, it may be useful to conceptualize individual and group identities as overlapping constructs which reinforce and redefine one another. Personal and collective identity and group identification were interrelated, and were important in the biographical work of negotiating the misalignment of identity upon entry to the new social world of HIV, and relating the new view of the self as HIV-positive to existing conceptions of the self and to others with HIV.

Seeking support and becoming a member of Helping Hand helped participants to realize their potential to change their lives and to become more active and confident with their HIV. Living with HIV involved adjustment to a new social world. Social worlds are groups which share resources, commitments, discourse, and a basis of collective action (Strauss 1993). Therefore, being able to relate in a meaningful way to others with HIV facilitated positive orientation to the new reality of HIV by enhancing access to resources through discourse. Rachel enjoyed time spent socializing with the other patients at the program and it allowed her to be a part of a community where she did not have to maintain the veil of secrecy regarding her HIV status. David felt that Helping Hand was instrumental in reducing his shame and discomfort in being seen at the clinic and that he became very active in the HIV community. Nancy described Helping Hand as beneficial, and related to the other HIV patients in an engaged manner, accepted her illness, and wanted to help others cope with their HIV. Involvement in support groups such as Helping Hand may be beneficial for HIV patients, facilitating positive group identification with the HIV-community, increasing access to resources such as information and relationships to similar others and reducing fear of stigma.

Similar to Walter, Chris, George, and Arthur did not discuss any membership in Helping Hand and did not seem to be active in the HIV-positive community. However, they seemed to accept their HIV and to have reconciled HIV with their self-view. Many of the participants displayed social personalities and emphasized having many friendships. However, sociability was expressed in relation to different reference groups. Walter related to the world of entertainment and music and because he denied that he had HIV he did not relate to people with HIV. Chris, George, and Arthur related to people with HIV but were highly selective in disclosure and perhaps because they felt healthy they did not feel the need to be immersed in the HIV-positive community. The worlds of work as a professional, family member, and being a part of the gay lifestyle were more relevant to them. Therefore, while sociability may play a role in seeking care and being involved in HIV services, it seemed that it was not necessarily if someone was social that determined their acceptance of care but rather to what groups someone related to and felt comfortable socializing with. Sense of belonging was enhanced when participants felt that others' life conditions and positions were relevant to their own life experiences and were consistent with their self-views. For Rachel, David, and Nancy the physical need for treatment brought them to the clinic, but after being referred to Helping Hand and developing a sense of belonging with the other Helping Hand members, they became more immersed in the HIV-positive community.

For example, before joining Helping Hand, Rachel would only come to see her physician and would not talk to the other patients. Interestingly, she said that this was what coming to the clinic was like for many of the patients. Rachel felt that the patients saw one another but did not want to get to know each other or to speak. But for Rachel this changed, she could now talk to the other patients, it no longer bothered her to talk to the other patients because she felt that "we are all the same" (Transcript 2, lines 361-362). Entering Helping Hand helped to redefine the way Rachel identified with the other patients and gave her access to membership in the HIV-positive community in a safe place where everyone was the same and she did not have to fear being identified as being different or being excluded. Therefore, both time spent living with HIV and HIV services served to ease PLWHA into a socially supportive group environment with others living with HIV, allowing them a safe place where they did not need to fear exclusion.

3.5.1.4   Compassionate Love

Another process structure of action was identified at the relational level. Giving and receiving compassionate love emerged as beneficial to coping with HIV. This is consistent with prior research which demonstrated that positive life changes can involve compassionate love which can improve well-being among people with HIV (Lutz et al. 2011). Compassionate love can be a driver for action, thus enabling agency. Compassionate love is a concept developed by Underwood (2008) which involves components of: freedom of choice, cognitive understanding, value-empowerment, openness and receptivity, response of the heart, concern, and action.

Compassionate love can be given or received. Because coping and social support are focal concepts of this analysis, compassionate love was a concept of interest. Social support can take many forms based on the type of support (instrumental versus emotional) and relationship (friend, family, intimate partner, physician) (Aneshensel 1992; Thoits 1995). Compassionate love can provide support to people by empowering them to take action to help themselves and others. Compassionate love is a relational concept because it is rooted in social relationships of care. Compassionate love can be viewed as distinct from social support because compassionate love involves a deep and loving commitment to care, and an awareness and understanding of the needs of the self and others.

Chris demonstrated a strong desire to help others and placed a high value on giving and receiving love. Love, helping others, and the empowerment gained from compassionate love helped Chris to take action and to maintain his identity as a social, positive, and likeable person. Identity and agency may play complementary roles, reinforcing one another and shaping the form and direction of action. Chris felt that his profession as a teacher provided him with a deep sense of meaning and empowerment:

> "Having this job as a teacher I help kids everyday I make them happy that means a lot to me (-) Um if I would have this disease and I wouldn't do anything good in my life I think I'd be feeling differently (-) like if I would just have to work at a factory like and do just stupid stuff like just like the same move over and over for eight hours like senseless to me (-) I could never do it I always wanted to be with people and touch people and help people." [Transcript 3, lines 304-308]

Chris felt that his job allowed him to help others on a daily basis; he was able to touch the lives of the children he worked with. Chris expressed a strong desire to give compassionate love, care, and support to others. Relationships of care and support were emphasized throughout his narrative. Chris felt that a profession that was removed from meaningful social interaction was "senseless" for him and expressed a deep need for meaningful relationships with others. Chris continued:

> "Even though that I'm sick um I still see good in it because with my personality (-) with just the things I do I can change the world. (-) like (-) you know (-) just by um being there for a kid that has no dad or that's not being treated well at home just by me spending time with them reading a book with them or like being silly and like tickling them (-) you know or just cuddling with them gives a lot (-) And um so (--) I get to live on with every person I meet (-) or actually every kid because I influence their life you know? And um that's really amazing (-) that's really amazing." [Transcript 3, lines 310-316]

Chris had a positive outlook on life and felt that with his personality and actions he could change the world by making a difference in each child's life. Giving support to children at his work was rewarding and allowed Chris to leave a legacy of giving. Touching other's lives in a meaningful way inspired and empowered Chris. Without the opportunity to have these interactions, Chris may not have been able to maintain an active lifestyle. This highlights the importance of preventing isolation and promoting meaningful and fulfilling interaction in order to encourage action and to overcome suffering. Giving compassionate love and leaving a legacy with each person Chris had a positive influence on was a major driving force in his life. Leaving a legacy allowed him to feel that he could "change the world." Chris was aware of the effect his own demeanor and actions had on the level of social interaction. Therefore, helping others through his profession empowered Chris and allowed him to be attuned to his personal sense of agency by feeling that he could change the world. Receiving love was also instrumental in empowerment. Chris described how he found true love and support:

> "It's really like helpful and really important I think if (-) if you have someone supportive in your life because (-) um like my partner he stood by me and said 'Well it doesn't affect me' and it turns out that he's positive too now and he said that 'I'll never blame you for anything' like 'I love you just as much' like he was really (-) really supportive and I have to say if it wouldn't have been for him (-) if I wouldn't have met him months earlier and he wouldn't have helped me through this actually I don't know how I would have responded to it (-) because I'm doing pretty well like I took it really good like there's not one day where I regret it or where I say 'I wish I could turn back time' because nothing has changed. Like I (-) I found real love (-) I found emotions (-) I found support (-) what I've always been looking for in a relationship and I haven't had before." [Transcript 3, lines 38-46]

Chris felt that his own experience of being supported and having a partner who loved and accepted him despite his diagnosis helped him to deal with his diagnosis. Chris may not have responded as actively to his HIV diagnosis if it was not for this loving, supportive relationship. Unconditional love and acceptance and having a partner to stand by Chris was instrumental in helping Chris resolve this moment of crisis, where he initially felt that his diagnosis also meant the end of his relationship. Chris felt that he coped with his diagnosis in a positive way. He did not have any regrets because he felt that nothing had changed. He was healthy and not currently on medication. Also, his diagnosis allowed him to experience "real love" and to find "emotions" and "support" which was what he had always searched for before and never experienced. The moment of crisis allowed Chris to experience true love because his partner accepted him and stood by him in his time of need and did not change the way he treated him. Chris elaborated:

> "Just knowing that the disease itself isn't that big of a deal like it was fifteen or twenty years ago so that second step that helped me was when I came here to the clinic and talked to the doctor and um he just told us straight out how it was and how it is (-) how it is these days and how it was back in the days he also mentioned there might be some side effects but um they weren't that big of a deal to me (-) maybe like a little dizziness or like yeah some people gain weight some people lose weight it comes and goes in all situations of life and I'm just not just by having HIV." [Transcript 3, lines 234-241]

Chris described steps in a process which helped him to negotiate his illness. First, it was his supportive relationship and the "second step" was obtaining information from the physicians at the clinic. Based on the information Chris received from the physician, he felt that HIV was not as big of an issue as it was in prior decades. The living conditions of HIV had changed and this seemed to reassure Chris. His physician discussed the side effects, such as dizziness or weight gain but these were not a major concern to Chris. Weight fluctuations were seen as normal and common instead of as a HIV-specific problem to Chris. Chris was healthy, not on medication, and was neither thin nor overweight. Perhaps he did not feel that weight was a major issue because his illness was not visible in his appearance. In contrast, Rachel experienced extensive weight loss, which she felt marked her as being sick and that caused considerable stress and discrimination. Chris said that weight change was not specific to HIV but later in the interview used appearance, specifically weight, as an indicator of determination of a person's HIV status. Chris explained the third support which helped him and elaborated on appearance:

> "I have um family who loves me even though they know I have HIV nothing has changed everything is still the same. I think that they tend to forget it also because it's not like something you see on the outside if someone has cancer and they go to chemotherapy and they lose their hair that's different you see it and so you suddenly get reminded and you might pity that person or you be like 'oh yeah um how are you doing?' but like I still look the same (-) I still talk the same so I think my family also forgets sometimes don't see it as that big of a deal." [Transcript 3, lines 243-252]

Chris felt that his family loved him despite his HIV status and that they treated him the same as before his diagnosis. However, he felt that his family forgot that he was HIV-positive because it was not externally visible. Chris compared HIV to cancer and felt that the treatment for cancer, chemotherapy, leaves a visible mark of illness (hair loss) which is a reminder of cancer that could induce pity or inquiries about illness. But Chris appeared and acted the same and so he felt that his family forgot that he had HIV and they treated him more normally and as a healthy person. Therefore, Chris recognized that appearance and the lack of visible sign or cues, such as thinness may influence how people viewed him and shaped his interactions. Interestingly, Chris discussed the media and entertainment. For Chris, the media communicated to him conceptions of beauty and sexual attractiveness. Chris discussed his struggle with maintaining a focus on internal substance and beauty in the context of his awareness of images of external beauty as he told:

> "I like to see the beautiful stuff inside of people that's important (-) and I always say like um if I end up sixty five or seventy and I look back on my like 'oh yeah great I've had a hot boyfriend and he was really popular and famous and a lot of money that's not gonna make me happy' like if I can look back and say 'Yeah I met this one person who loves me truly for who I am and for what I am and um I feel the same' that's what's most important for me and if that person I met that time um was so supportive by just loving me so it gave me the feeling that even if I have to die in a month or two like I'm not really afraid because I found what I've been looking for so long (-) like emotions and someone who loves me and that is um (-) that in itself is more beautiful than any money or any person can ever be you know?" [Transcript 3, lines 221-229]

For Chris, it was the beauty within people that was truly important and his distinction between internal and external beauty or reality demonstrated how he made sense of his social world and formulated his view of reality. Chris explained if he were to reflect back on his life in the future it would be meaningless for him to say that he had been with an attractive, popular, rich, and famous man because these things did not make him truly happy. Instead, if Chris could one day reflect upon his life and say that he had experienced true, unconditional love that was what was most meaningful for him. Receiving love and support gave Chris the strength to face the possibility of death and to decide to have no fear because he had found the love he had been seeking in this life. Finding true love and acceptance took away his fear of death and made Chris feel that even if he should have to face death, he could do so knowing that he had found what he had always been searching for. Chris continued:

> "Even though I tend to forget it a lot of times because you just get hit with all these shallow things around you like commercials and this and that 'You have to look like this and like that' and of course I go with it and I go to the gym and I try to look my best too you know it's not like that but that helped me to get through" [Transcript 3; lines 231-234].

Interestingly, Chris expressed turmoil as he reported that he often forgot the importance of inner beauty and true love because he was affected by the shallow representations in the media that told him that he must look a certain way in order to be attractive. Chris valued inner beauty but also had to face the superficial, surface images of beauty in the media, which he conformed to by taking care to go to the gym and to "look his best." Appearance was a theme which emerged again later in the interview when Chris discussed stigma. Chris felt that appearance could grant acceptance and normality if one fit the image of beauty expected in society.

Both Walter and Chris received information and images from the media and processed this information in an active manner. Walter placed a high value on truth and looking beneath the surface representations in the media to reveal the truth, which he felt existed underneath the external. Chris valued beauty but struggled with superficial or external images of beauty and the internal beauty that he felt truly was important in life. Themes of looking beneath the surface or external in order to reveal what was meaningful emerged for both Chris and Walter. Chris actively tried to maintain a focus on inner beauty, while Walter actively resisted images of the media and critically evaluated them in order to determine the truth hidden amongst the illusions in entertainment. True love and beauty empowered Chris to maintain a positive outlook and to maintain control over his life.

The importance of love and relationships of care was also emphasized in the Miami sample. Being involved in support groups sometimes had other benefits such as finding love and starting new intimate relationships. Giving up on love after HIV diagnosis was reported in both samples. Participants often felt that HIV would destroy their existing partnerships or prevent them from forming new intimate relationships. Participants in both samples reported finding love after HIV but this was a complicated issue. Some participants reported dating different partners at different times and the process of finding love took time and was not easy. Finding love and acceptance was important and helped participants to feel accepted and supported. In addition, being part of an intimate and loving relationship appeared to grant participants with a sense of normalcy in the face of a strange, new life. By having a partner and also by having children, participants appeared to gain a sense of normalcy and belonging.

Similar to the Frankfurt sample, Miami participants reported that their children were a source of support. Interestingly, social support from children was also discussed as an exchange, where interviewees had to provide reassurance and support to their children, while at the same time feeling cared for and loved by their children. Giving love and care to children and grandchildren emerged as helpful in the face of adversity but was not without its own challenges and concerns. However, overall participants described that providing, loving, and caring for others enabled them go on in the face of HIV. Living to see children make important life events such as graduating from school was a major driver for participants. When faced with the initial diagnosis of HIV, and as they learned to deal with HIV in daily life as a chronic illness, participants drew on social support to help them to feel strong and continue to move forward in their daily lives to maintain a healthy and productive mindset.

3.5.1.5   Giving Social Support and Helping Others

Helping others emerged as an important aspect of participants' lives in the Miami sample. Interestingly, while social demands were reported among the participants, helping others also emerged as a positive experience, enhancing feelings of empowerment and efficacy. Similar to the Frankfurt sample, participants in the Miami sample derived a great sense of meaning, purpose, and strength by helping others. Giving social support and helping others helped to reduce feelings of social isolation and to enhance social integration and sense of belonging.

Conceptualizations of social support can be limited by overlooking the context-bound conditions of biographical adjustment to HIV and the processes involved in giving and receiving care. For example, depending on when people were asked, their reports of social support were more or less pronounced due to the social context of their lives. Also, issues which can be process-based, such as issues in the effective timing of receiving support, could be affected by the timing of interviews. Support must also be desired, pursued, and fitting to the social positions, needs, and social characteristics of patients. Research on social support could be improved by integrating concepts reflecting the processes involved in social support, such as those of group identification and by assessing contextual and procedural issues encountered when seeking and obtaining support such as temporal, spatial, and financial constraints.

3.5.1.6   Relations of Care and Social Support: Emotional and Financial Resources

Social support helped to facilitate positive outcomes such as thriving, improved relations to self and others, acceptance of HIV, and engagement in healthy, productive behavior among participants. Social support has been defined as "functions performed for the individual by significant others, such as family members, friends, and coworkers. Significant others can provide instrumental, informational, and/or emotional assistance" (House and Kahn 1985 as discussed in Thoits 1995). Perceived emotional support is defined as the belief that significant others are available to provide "love and caring, sympathy and understanding, and/or esteem and value" (Thoits 1995). Emotional support, especially in reaction to HIV disclosure, can help to enhance feelings of acceptance and to reduce stress. For example, participants discussed the importance of emotional support and feeling loved and cared for or having someone in their life who they believed understood their needs and affirmed their sense of self-worth. Friends were a valuable source of support.

Importantly, being involved in social support groups was reported as helpful by participants and provided a safe place to exchange ideas, information, and experiences with HIV. However, in the process of receiving social support, participants reported issues in seeking support. Seeking social support was an important factor in establishing positive and empowering relationships with others in the face of adversity. After seeking support, social support should be timely, effective, and meet people's expectations. Institutional barriers and procedural issues needed to be minimized in order to enable effective and efficient support.

Social support was part of a process of taking action that was process- and context-based. The social context of social support affected the quality of support and its effectiveness as a resource. Also, different sources of support could provide different forms of support (Primomo et al. 1990). Primomo and colleagues (1990) found that among women with chronic illness, that women report more social support from a partner than from family, friends, or others and that family members were a source of affective support whereas friends provide feelings of affirmation. Others suggest that components of social support including: amount, timing, source, structure, and function of support can influence how social support shapes mental health outcomes (Shinn et al. 1984). However, such studies are often divorced from biographical experience. The current analysis, which is grounded in life experience and social meaning, demonstrates how social context can create conditions that contextualize the experience of giving and receiving social support. Compassionate love and social support emerged as distinct but overlapping concepts in this analysis. Although both compassionate love and social support were related to relationships of care and to giving and receiving care, compassionate love emerged as a distinct concept which involved a deep, emotional connection to the self and to others. Compassionate love had a transformative potential and this emerged as being associated with participants' relationships with children.

3.5.1.7   Children and Compassionate Love

Children were discussed as a source of giving and receiving compassionate love. Rachel had two sons who she conceived after she was diagnosed and who were born HIV-negative due to her careful adherence to medical regimens. Rachel discussed her children as being instrumental to her well-being and providing a valuable feeling of support and structure to her life as she explained:

> "Before I had children I was (-) I was alone (-) my mom was going to work and I stay alone the whole day (-) that was really (-) not good (-) yeah (-) but now since I have children they can go and a day will end without (-) without thinking about that I'm sick (-) yeah (-) Cause I have to do this (-) do this (-) do the other (-) go to the children to play outside and then at the end of the day I'm tired and sleep." [Transcript 2, lines 436-444]

Nancy reported a similar experience of feeling alone before having her children and emphasized the importance of having children throughout her narrative. Nancy went through a series of attempts to become pregnant safely after her HIV diagnosis and experienced a miscarriage during this process. The experience of her miscarriage served to initiate a positive turning point in Nancy's life. Similar to Rachel, Nancy explained that the reason she wanted to get pregnant was because she always felt alone she "Wanted to have a partner, someone who would just share everything with me, my body, my blood, everything" (Sequential Report 6, p. 2). When Nancy went to the doctor and the doctor told her the baby's heart was not beating she was devastated. Nancy had to have the baby aborted and go the same day for her driver's license exam. She passed the driving exam and she said that this was "the beginning of her good life" (Sequential Report 6, p. 3). Nancy explained that "it was like a good thing happened and a bad thing happened" in the same day. Nancy lost her child and she told herself she wasn't going to push it anymore and decided to relax and to take care of herself (Sequential Report 6, p. 3).

Nancy explained getting pregnant was very difficult because it required her and her husband to take sperm and put it into a syringe and push it into her body. The process to have a child was very difficult and she stopped trying to have a baby. Eventually, Nancy tried to get pregnant again and was successful; she had to go to the doctor many times throughout her pregnancy to take care of her unborn child and he was born HIV-negative. The birth of Nancy's son gave her hope that life could still be normal. Four years later, Nancy got pregnant again. This pregnancy to her was amazing because she was not trying to get pregnant and also because it turned out that she was pregnant with twins. Nancy was afraid but told herself to fight, that she had fought the virus before, and had a child before, that she used to go to doctors to get injections so that she could get pregnant and this pregnancy happened so easily, that God had given her this pregnancy.

Having twins was a shock to Nancy because she was HIV-positive, even one child was more than she would have ever expected. The twins were born about a week early. When Nancy gave birth even though she was operated on she wanted to watch the twin's birth. For Nancy, this pregnancy was like a story and she wanted to see the end of it because she could not believe she was having twins with her HIV. Nancy watched each child's birth, one minute after the other, and they were healthy. This gave her hope. Her life became brighter. At the time of the interview, Nancy had three children at home and all children were healthy. Having children was very important to Nancy and gave her hope for a normal life and for companionship. Nancy felt supported by her children and that her children gave her strength. Nancy described how every day she would look at her children and tell herself "I have something to live for, I have my children to live for, and my children give me strength" (Sequential Report 6, p. 6).

Sarah also felt that her children were a source of support and love. Sarah had her children before she was diagnosed with HIV. Sarah waited over a decade to disclose her HIV status to her children because she chose to wait until her children were of the age of eighteen. Sarah described her experience disclosing to her children:

"Oh it wasn't easy at all (-) of course not (-) I mean (exhales) but this was somehow the (-) the aim for myself or the (-) I had told to myself in the beginning 'I won't tell them anything before they're adults' and can understand that better or can deal with that better (-) in a better way (-) that's why I waited until they were (--) you have to find some time and that was (-) for me (-) it was eighteen (-) and well it was a big shock of course (-) hearing your mother is ill (-) probably deadly ill (-) this is the association problem that you have as far as (-) ah the second thing is the all the other thoughts associated with that (-) 'How come your mother got that?' (changes tone of voice) (-) 'So what about your father?' 'What was he like?' HIV is connected with homosexuality so they also had to have to think that thought." [Transcript 5, lines 317-326]

Sarah had a great consideration of the potential emotional impact of her HIV disclosure to her children, which was displayed by her waiting until they reached adulthood to disclose when she felt they would be more mature and able to handle this information. She described this as a shock to her children and this shock appeared to be anticipated. She put herself in her children's perspectives and tried to construct their thought process and how this would lead to questions about their father and the nature of their father's character and sexuality. Once Sarah's children knew about her HIV their reaction was very supportive. However, the topic of the father was taboo. No one wanted to discuss the implications for the father's character and sexuality due to Sarah's HIV. Sarah described their relationship:

> "We have a very special relationship (-) again (-) I don't think our relationship is as good because of the HIV (-) probably we would have the same good relationship anyway (-) […] they are very empathetic (-) you know (-) and very (-) really both of them very thoughtful (-) very caring."

When asked if this was a comfort Sarah responded affirmatively:

> "Of course (-) of course (-) It is one of the main factors and so I make it as long as I did."
> [Transcript 5, lines 361-368]

Sarah's relationship with her children was instrumental in Sarah's survival and ongoing effort to maintain control over her life. Receiving unconditional love and understanding comforted Sarah in her day to day life and helped her to remain strong and to press on. Indeed, when Sarah described her reaction to her own HIV diagnosis she emphasized the importance of her children:

> "The world didn't break down because I had two little children so that was first of all (-) the (--) decision you have to go through that (-) you have to make it (-) somehow." [Transcript 5, lines 33-35]

Sarah felt a need to keep her world intact so that she could take care of her children. The holding of her world together was a conscious decision that she had to "go through" in order to care for her children. The strong commitment she had to her role as a caregiver to her children indicated that her engagement in a committed relationship of care served to stabilize her in a moment of existential crisis on the brink of disorder. This demonstrated that her commitment to maintain her relationship with her children helped to provide her with a sense of coherence and stability in the face of the existential crisis of HIV.

3.5.2   *Transformational Biographical Processes*

3.5.2.1   Psychoanalysis as Creative Metamorphosis of Identity

Transformational biographical processes emerged in both the Frankfurt and Miami samples. Here, the process of creative metamorphosis of identity is discussed. Sarah provided a clear case of this process, her psychoanalysis served as a creative metamorphosis identity process structure facilitating self-discovery and empowerment:

> "I had a psychotherapy a long one started with a so-called 'immediate intervention' which is twenty five hours and that was very good of course and after that we turned that into a psychoanalysis (-) I had a psychoanalysis which lasted about six years (-) it was a Freudian analysis (-) and well I think that was the most helpful thing about it (-) all this personal (--) ah strength (-) and uh you know (-) the will (-) or (-) or the personality itself this (-) this psychoanalysis was the biggest support (-) or the biggest reason also for (-) for all these things being successful." [Transcript 5, lines 124-137]

Sarah sought out psychotherapy as a means to cope with her challenges and this process lasted six years. Sarah felt that the most helpful benefit of her psychoanalysis was the personal strength that she realized within in her "will" or "personality." The strength she found in herself via psychoanalysis was a major source of support and she felt this support from her psychoanalysis was the most important factor in her coming to terms with her HIV. Sarah was a Turkish woman who had been living in Germany for a long period of time. It was unclear when her family first came to Germany. Sarah sought out a therapeutic method that takes a great deal of time and commitment to be effective, which suggested that Sarah felt a deep need to continue this type of therapy. I probed and asked her more about her psychoanalysis and she explained:

> "I have an interest in Psychology and Psychiatry and Psychoanalysis all the time anyway (-) and so I'd been reading a lot (-) so I didn't just jump into the cold water (-) I knew what I was doing (-) and after having had this psychotherapy (-) at the beginning (-) it was just sitting (-) it wasn't normal psychotherapy (-) And then my doctor (-) my analyst asked me what about (-) if I could imagine having a psychoanalysis and so on and I said 'Ok let's go ahead a try it' and it was ok (-) so I did that for at least six years (-) I mean you always have breaks and holidays and all this that's why it takes so long (-) And (-) but there were times where I had to come to Frankfurt three times a week and with the small children it wasn't (-) probably not very easy (-) at that time I probably didn't really realize it (-) but uh but I went working all the time (-) I never stopped working." [Transcript 5, lines 139-168]

Sarah displayed a deep commitment and interest in psychotherapy as she explained that she had a strong interest in Psychology and sought out her treatment after seeking information about psychotherapy. Sarah also displayed a highly active character at this time in her life. She traveled from her home in a small town to Frankfurt three times a week as she was also working and taking care of her young children. Sarah emphasized her feeling of acting in the moment and being in the present situation, which made events acute and focused her attention so that she acted without taking the time to stop. She felt that only twenty years later she had gotten a bit slower because her life circumstances no longer forced her to function at such a high level of activity because her children were older and could care for themselves.

Sarah reflected on her past situation as she said "Now looking back I say 'Gee, you made it.' (laughs) It wasn't easy probably" and described that she was also tired at that time or must have been. The manner in which she described this experience suggests that she thought in a very needs-based, automated way at that time because her daily routine and responsibilities were so demanding that looking back in time she could reflect on how it must have been hard, she must have been tired. But this moment was long behind her and her thoughts of her effort and the potential stress and fatigue in maintaining such an active lifestyle were minimized. Sarah said that she never complained to anyone, not even to herself about the difficulty of her situation, she simply pressed on, which demonstrated a strong resolve and deep commitment to her well-being and survival.

Interestingly, psychoanalysis was a very reflective process and Sarah told that she simply acted in the situation and did not take time to think and yet was spending a substantial amount of time every week undergoing a deeply introspective therapy. Perhaps psychoanalysis allowed her to process her emotions in a more cognitively conscious way so that she could regulate her emotions more easily and cope with her life circumstances. Indeed, throughout the interview, Sarah was open but also very cerebral, which suggests that she experienced her emotions, but by processing them in a systematic and intellectual way, she may at the same time distance herself from emotional pain by focusing on the processing and regulation of her emotions rather than feeling the full thrust of her emotional content. I asked more about her psychoanalysis and Sarah responded:

"You do encounter some sort of uh well (-) I wouldn't say change of personality but somehow uh you get your possibilities (-) your talents (-) or you realize about yourself (-) you find yourself maybe (-) that's it (-) I could name it like that (-) yes (-) you dig yourself out from somewhere

and then you find some way and then since then (--) I do recommend it to anyone (-) to anyone (laughs) I say if it was for me I would make it obligatory for anyone after (uv) at least to have them do it once (-) and yes (-) so (-) of course I'm enthusiastic about that so and uh three (-) no two years ago I didn't (-) I wasn't (-) there was also some (-) in that summer (-) I had very much stress probably and that summer my little one was finishing gymnasium the older one was finishing his uh vocational training (-) It was a stressful time (-) and that was more than ten years after I had finished my analysis (-) but I called my analyst and was thinking 'how about (-) can you give me an appointment?' 'Of course (-)' and immediately we started again that was like a psychotherapy again now (-) once a week (-) only once a week (-) but it was very helpful."
[Transcript 5, lines 171-185]

Sarah used psychotherapy to cope with her stress. Sarah linked her stress to her children's educational careers and turning points in the life course. When Sarah felt oncoming stress, she took action to contact her therapist immediately and to continue her psychotherapy. Interestingly, she described the process of her inner discovery of her strength. Sarah described a biographical process of self-discovery of her potential and talent, which was part of finding herself. She described finding herself as "digging" herself from somewhere and then finding a way to continue on and to utilize her strength. Sarah's engagement in psychoanalysis resembled the biographical process structure of creative metamorphosis as proposed by Schütze (2007):

"Creative metamorphoses of biographical identity by which a new important inner development is starting in one's own biography, that might be miraculous and irritating in the beginning since it is new and that initially prohibits pertinent competencies of the biography incumbent, and towards which she or he must find out what the very quality of it might be." (p. 11 f.)

Furthermore, Schütze posited that creative metamorphosis also involves:

"The relationship of biographical metamorphosis between the identity of the biography incumbent and social processes is characterized by the attitude of encountering and exploring something essentially new in a social encounter and especially in one's biographical identity and life history, which is not conditioned by outer forces and normative expectation pattern, but stems from the inner identity realm of the biography incumbent and/or her or his interaction partners. A basic feature of the attitude of the metamorphosis relationship is the orientation structure of being puzzled by the dynamics of inner change of one's personal or of individual identity and of feeling driven to find out what are the riddles of it." (p. 23)

Sarah encountered a new aspect of her identity, her inner strength, by engaging in this reflexive process of psychoanalysis with her therapist as her identity partner as she explored her inner world. Sarah was driven to pursue this process from the moment she decided to seek therapy. Her drive to undergo this process was indicated by her seeking information and reading about psychotherapy, her selective choice of a therapist, and the constant effort in daily life over the years to travel to the city in order to undergo this process even though she was both working and caring for her children. Therefore, Sarah engaged in substantial biographical work in her psychotherapy as she delved deep into herself and her experiences to realize her potential and to regain her connection with her true self. This process was integral to her negotiation of HIV as she felt that it was the biggest factor in her success. Sarah's process of deep, reflexive self-discovery enabled her to become attuned with her agency, aware of her strength, and to come to terms with her HIV.

Therefore, identity and action can be intertwined at different levels. In the case of Helping Hand, action and identity were rooted in the social-contextual and relational aspects of individual and collective identity and group identification as participants related to others. At the biographical and internal level, creative metamorphosis of identity contributed to the development of action. By identifying and fortifying the self and caring for her children, Sarah was able to find her inner strength and to realize her human potential and agency.

Agency may thus be conceptualized as involving multiple processes and conditions at different levels of experience. The debate of agency as a micro versus macro phenomena can potentially be resolved by focusing on a more refined analysis of the development of agency as involving numerous intermediate processes at different levels of social reality and experience. Indeed, Giddens (1995) proposed an interactionist view of human agency, where structure and agency were conceptualized as interdependent and linked by strategic action. Therefore, understanding strategic action as rooted in multi-level processes can refine conceptualizations of agency and action. Because action emerged in this analysis at multiple levels of social reality and experience, biographical methods facilitated an understanding of how social-contextual, relational, and biographical level processes were related to action. Creativity, action, and transformative processes were important in biographical adjustment to HIV.

3.5.2.2   Creative Production, Innovation, and Entrepreneurship

Creative production can enhance feelings of inspiration, increasing drive and empowering people to be active and to embark on further creative and productive enterprises. Engaging in creative production (channeling energy and taking action to develop creative and productive projects) and entrepreneurship (organizing, developing, and managing new business ventures) appeared to be empowering and a source of vitality in the face of illness among the Miami sample. Creative work was identified as a biographical process structure of action which occurred on the biographical level. Creative work also extended to the relational level as people collaborated on projects and extended their work outside of themselves and into the working world. Escaping a trajectory of suffering can involve creativity as Riemann and Schütze (1991) posited:

> "The overwhelming and long-lasting process of suffering gives the person the chance of systematic reflection, of finding a deep relationship to her- or himself and to the world and to significant others, and of mobilizing biographical work and creativity. This can be followed by well-organized biographical action schemes for controlling the dynamics of disorder and by the exploration and development of hitherto unseen personal capabilities, that is, by a creative metamorphosis of the state of biographical identity." (p. 343 f.)

Some participants in Miami described their involvement in a number of creative projects that served to motivate and inspire them. Unlike Walter who did not use his music to inform about HIV, some participants used their creativity and to increase awareness of HIV. This was an important aspect of this type of action process structure because the product of creative production had the potential to influence other's views of HIV in the public. Creative production enhanced action on a personal and biographical level as it inspired and motivated participants to be active and to have aspirations, inspiration, and goals, but also extended to an even higher level of influence as they collaborated with other professionals to put their projects into action. In Frankfurt, David was active in trying to increase awareness of HIV. However, David was not open about his HIV status and media coverage of David's activism revealed his HIV status without his consent. Being open about HIV posed a risk but also allowed participants access to support. Participants in Miami discussed being active in their efforts to develop their projects as they networked with other professionals and worked to cultivate creative inspiration to create momentum and meaning in their lives.

Importantly, to fund creative projects participants discussed working other jobs that were described as monotonous and that were not intellectually demanding to provide them with the financial resources needed to fund their true passions. While it is difficult to determine whether most Americans work in a similar style, it is likely that this approach to work would be more common among creative and entrepreneur type professionals who have the opportunities and drive to work in multiple fields, and who lack the funding they require to pursue their passions. The lack of sufficient financial means to support the pursuit of entrepreneurial and creative projects was described as contributing to a sense of strain. Creative production appeared to involve biographical work affected by conditions of financial resources. In a context of limited financial resources, strain emerged in maintaining the continuous effort, commitment, and dedication needed to engage in entrepreneurial work. This strain could be especially heightened in the context of a global recession and weakening of the American economy.

Because a foundational aspect of innovation is creativity, the action participants took to create new businesses can be conceptualized as an act of creative production. In the absence of programs that people felt were suitable to fit the needs of people with HIV, a participant mobilized to launch an organization that provided these services. Others engaged in HIV activism or other artistic projects to raise awareness about HIV. Giving support to the HIV-positive community after a HIV diagnosis was discussed as empowering. It is also possible that because patients in Frankfurt had access to the support services in Helping Hand, unlike the Miami participants they did not have to mobilize to create alternate sources of support because innovation requires creating alternative solutions in the absence of support.

Facilitating social relationships was an important aspect of providing support to others. Women with children expressed the desire to inform HIV-positive people about their experiences successfully having HIV-negative children. Prior to engagement in personally meaningful work and social activities, participants often felt emotionally disconnected from others, suggesting a sense of anomie (Merton 1938). Innovation was discussed by Merton (1938) as a mode of adaptation to strain which involved the rejection of culturally acceptable means but acceptance of cultural goals as it related to the commission of crime. However, the channeling of action into new enterprises which do not violate the prevailing social laws as described by the participants in this study, suggests that creative responses to strain can contain elements of rebellion as described by Merton (1938) by creating new opportunities and professions, which do not completely overthrow the existing social order but which are innovative responses that create new opportunities and can change some elements of local context by raising awareness about social issues. Merton (1938) emphasized that the modes of adaptation to strain were rooted in personal experience and context and examining creative production, innovation, and entrepreneurship as a process of action rooted in personal biography highlighted the importance of personal history in adaptation to strain. Creative production could also represent rebellion as an adaptation to strain because, as described by participants, people's goals may also change based on their life experiences (Merton 1938). For those who described transformative change after their HIV diagnosis, their goals shifted from being based in the pursuit of material wealth to goals which centered on improving the welfare of others and that helped them emotionally connect to the world. Participants described a shift from individualistic goals such as fulfilling hedonistic desires in the form of drug use, sex, and material objects towards striving to contribute to a collective wealth. Therefore, creative production can correspond to Merton's (1938) description of rebellion where people reject cultural means and goals and create new means and goals. The expression of the form of creative production and entrepreneurial endeavors was deeply embedded in personal biography.

Importantly, transitions of both entering and exiting transformative and action processes structures were emphasized in the interviews. Despite efforts to combat stigma and raise awareness about HIV by being open about HIV status among those who were open about their HIV status, they also withdrew. Some withdrew from activities in their local religious communities and others withdrew from their businesses and HIV activism. The narratives contained the ongoing fundamental tensions in people's lives and the constellations of events that contributed in decisions to withdraw.

Diagnosis, disclosure, and adjustment to HIV cannot be reduced to singular concepts that lack grounding in personal experience, social meaning, and the constellation of events in personal history as they occur over time in historical context. Just as trajectories of suffering can be overcome so also can people exit action schemes when overwhelmed by their life experiences. Theoretical insights can be identified and developed by understanding the transitions between entries and exits from one biographical process to another. In this study, stressful life events such as the deaths of loved ones, persistent poverty, discrimination, and a lack of support were related to decisions to no longer be open about HIV status.

Notably, some participants also had manic depression, a mental health condition characterized by periods of intense and manic activity followed by an emotional crash characterized by depression and lethargy. Interestingly, those with manic depression exhibited remarkable productivity, creativity, and transformative change. Because manic depression represents a more dramatic shift in productivity and emotional states of euphoria and depression, the shifts between trajectories of suffering into biographical action process structures could have been more pronounced. Periods of intense productivity followed by exhaustion are not a phenomenon unique to only those with manic depression and could be more common especially in the current economic context in America, which has greatly destabilized the economic well-being of millions of Americans.

Interviewees in Frankfurt discussed seeking support but none defined themselves as having a mental illness. This difference may have been due to the research project in Miami being based in a Department of Psychology. Staff and students in the research center took detailed case notes of mental health issues and this may explain this difference. While beyond the scope of the current study, future research is encouraged to examine the ways that people experiencing similar health problems such as HIV conceptualize their emotions and cope with stress

The successes and exceptional transformative changes emergent in the narratives of those with manic depression suggest that what is socially constructed as a disease or mental illness is deeply rooted in biography. The intense bouts of productivity and inspiration could have been fueled by manic depression suggesting that conditions that are negatively valued in society can actually have deep, positive meanings for those who possess them despite their own suffering and can become a meaningful part of the self and action. However, more research is needed on how conditions such as manic depression relate to biography and intersect with other social positions and affect biography. It is possible that the distinct cultural contexts influenced how mental health problems were defined and treated by participants. For example, the medicalization of American society and widespread use of psychiatric medications to treat conditions such as depression and anxiety is distinct from that of other nations. PLWHA face unique challenges and understanding how mental health problems are treated has implications for their HIV treatment. Research examining how HAART and psychiatric medications could potentially interact in the body could be important for improving patient care.

3.5.2.3 Spirituality: HIV as a Spiritual Journey

Throughout their interviews, participants described numerous changes including changes in world view and of the spiritual. One aspect of their worldview and spirituality pertained to their view of God/higher power in the face of illness. Views of organized religion, spiritual entities, omnipresent beings, and of God/higher power appeared to be related to their views of humanity and their treatment by others in both a religious institutional context, and in the broader context of their lives. Reactions by others to HIV disclosure may be fundamental in shaping conceptions of humanity, society, and God. For example, exclusion and social distance by members of religious institutions can correspond with a view of God as punishing and not forgiving rather than a conception of God as accepting. Prior research suggests that conceptions of God are important in shaping health outcomes among people living with HIV (Kremer et al. 2009). Developing a supportive relationship with God and the spiritual was reported as important in developing feelings of agency and acceptance of HIV.

Struggles in relationships with God, religion, and sexual identity were inter-related. Conceptions of sexuality, sin, and HIV played an important role in how some participants viewed themselves and came to terms with their sexuality and HIV. Resolving this conflict and establishing a relationship with God and a positive self-view was instrumental in helping people to cope with their HIV and to maintain positive life changes. Discussions of feeling feel closed to God and feeling inadequate to God emerged in this analysis. Overcoming a faith based in fear was described as critical in opening to the spiritual. Learning about HIV and developing a sense of belonging with the HIV-positive community helped participants to resolve spiritual struggles and to stop destructive behavior.

Developing an understanding that one's relationship with God was personal and not to be defined by others emerged as important to overcoming a fear of God and a fear of change. The realization that the spiritual transcended ownership and that no one could legitimize a moral claim of ownership over the spiritual was a part of the process of resolving spiritual struggle. When wrestling with the problematized nature of sexuality and religion, feelings of unworthiness of God's love were barriers to self-acceptance. Learning to be true to one's self and making decisions that were aligned with one's personal conceptions of morality was related to creating a strong foundation of support and positivity. A HIV diagnosis was discussed as facilitating a change in beliefs and self-realization, such as resolving feelings of fear and hatred. Inner turmoil was rooted in other's conceptions of race/ethnicity and sexuality. Awareness of racism and discrimination towards gays contributed to a painful self-doubt as some participants integrated other's perspectives into their self-concepts. Letting go of the pain of discrimination based on sexuality and race/ethnicity was related to exiting self-destructive patterns of thoughts and behavior. Importantly, when participants internalized negative attitudes of others, this became a self-fulfilling prophecy and perpetuated feelings of worthlessness. Breaking this cycle of labeling was critical in restoring feelings of self-worth, relationships with the spiritual, and changing destructive behavior. Labeling emerged as a highly reflexive process in this analysis.

Accordingly, labeling can affect self-concept and behavior. Stigma can affect identity, sense of belonging, action, agency, emotions, and behavior. This indicates the importance of the intersectionality of race and sexuality because these personal struggles were rooted in multiple social positions. Also, some participants reported that although they were not religious they were still spiritual. View of humanity appeared to be related to view of religion because when participants felt they could not trust others and had negative views of humanity, they tended to distance themselves from organized religion and to not trust religious doctrines. Religious conceptions of gayness as sin were related to preferences of gay participants to develop their personal approaches to the spiritual rather than being involved in organized religion. Feelings towards religion and the nature of the spiritual and of humanity were rooted in biographical experience. In the Miami narratives, there were reports of abuse in childhood by religious figures. Experiencing abuse was related to the rejection of religion. Overcoming personal struggles with organized religion was an important aspect of the process of reestablishing a positive relationship and sense of belonging with the spiritual and with sexuality.

In a context of uncertainty and drastic life change, people may turn to religion as a form of support, but spiritual engagement was rooted in biographical experience and often involved elements of existential struggle. Turning to the spiritual for support may be motivated by a number of motives, such as a need for meaning, coherence, strength, and hope. However, experiences of discrimination and treatment by others that is cruel, alienating, and which poses a deep violation of the self can alter conceptions of both religious institutions and of the higher powers they are intended to represent as being unaccepting, cruel, judgmental, and even as being nihilistic and nonexistent. It is not the issue of whether there is an actual existence of a higher power that is the issue at hand. The issue is the perception of an existence of a higher power and the meaning which people link to such entities and the institutions that represent them. These views of God and religion can also reinforce a negative cycle whereby conceptions of God have serious implications for views of the self. A view of God as judgmental and unaccepting can reinforce a negative identity of the self as unworthy of the spiritual and of society. The spiritual can provide a grounds for a "looking glass self" (Cooley 1902).

When participants' lifestyles ran counter the religious doctrines of socially acceptable behavior and violated religious conceptions of morality, struggles with unworthiness and religiosity were emphasized. Feeling rejected by religious institutions was discussed as contributing to feelings of loneliness and social isolation. Religious rejection effectively restricted access to social capital and support available in religious institutions, and was felt as unjust and hypocritical. This suggests that having a religious institution that is welcoming, and that sincerely accepts and encourages people from all walks of life to be a part of its gatherings, can make a difference in people's lives. Feeling unworthy and not having a sense of belonging can prevent people from having a place where they can express themselves and be attuned to their spiritualty and to relate to others. Resolving religious conflicts and developing spirituality helped participants to be attuned with their agency and to press on in the face of adversity.

The location of religious institutions in relation to health care centers and participants' homes was discussed. For example, a participant discussed visiting a local church while waiting for medical treatment. This suggests that the location of institutions could be systemically targeted by urban planning and health care initiatives to improve patient care. The proximity of community health centers to religious organizations and other support services could facilitate ease of use and coordination of care. For PLWHA in segregated and impoverished communities, proximity of health care and support services to one another and to patient's neighborhoods could create an important context of their care based in location to ease the burden of seeking support.

Both intra- and inter-religious struggles were discussed. Resolving conflicts between different religious belief systems was important in developing a sense of connection and belonging to the spiritual that transcended social boundaries. Synthesizing religious beliefs created an even stronger overall view of the spiritual. Themes of immersion into a new culture and religion, and making meaningful connections between belief systems, cultures, and events emerged in this analysis. Themes of immersion into culture and religion were discussed in the context of music. Immersion into music and developing a deep sense of connection to the suffering of others through music as a means of belonging was discussed in the Miami sample. The development of spirituality was related to feelings of interconnectedness between mind, body, and spirit in conceptions of health and healing. In this analysis spirituality, which was discussed as the personal development of a meaningful relationship with the spiritual and which involved resolving religious conflicts emerged as an action process structure. Through spiritual growth, participants reconciled different belief systems, integrated their self-concepts in an accepting way with their belief systems, and established meaningful relationships with God or a higher power. Spiritual growth involved developing a sense of belonging and connection with the spiritual.

Seeking guidance from God or a higher power can be a form of seeking social support or spiritual support. As with other forms of social support, spiritual support can be seen as a process involving: 1. needs/conditions to desire support, 2. awareness of need/desire to seek support, 3. taking action to seek and obtain support, where the 4. context of support seeking shapes the effectiveness of support obtained and 5.effectiveness of support influenced further attempts and involvement in religious institutions and spiritual coping, and where this process is rooted in biographical context. People could work to establish a sense of belonging with the spiritual because of many and simultaneous needs. For example, asking God for forgiveness and asking God for help were important factors involved in views of God and spiritual support processes. Emotional conflicts grounded in moral discourse could complicate spiritual support seeking and conceptions of God, such as feeling closed to or angry at God, unworthy, or of an ultimate rejection of institutions and their religious doctrines.

Conceptions of God/higher power appeared to be related to views of a higher power's intention in regards to meaning making of HIV. When wrestling with the question "Why do I have HIV?" interviewees constructed various answers to make sense of their diagnosis. Some participants reported a view of God giving them HIV as a form of hardship that could allow them to help others. Others also reported a belief that God was giving them what they were able to handle. Some even expressed a sense of gratitude to God. Meaning making was complex and occurred in the context of interconnected beliefs, which involved conceptions of God's nature, God's intention, and the purpose of being chosen to live with HIV. These beliefs appeared to be related to attitudes towards God, which were positive (such as gratitude) and attitudes about the self as powerful, able to help others, and filled with purpose and intention in society. Spiritual experiences such as visualizations of communicating with nature and heavenly beings emerged in the Miami narratives.

These visions transcended the bounds of language and involved heavenly beings of a transcendental nature that existed beyond the culturally defined symbols of communication. This transcendence suggests a deep sense of longing for a connection and belonging to the universe. Visions of animals, nature, and spiritual beings and were described as involving receiving messages from God, to express God's love and generosity, and to prepare for adversity to come. Abstractions are creations of the mind when making sense of experience. The construction of these visions can thus be deconstructed in order to further understand how participants constructed their views of reality. The visions described often involved animals or heavenly creatures and not other human beings, and may have represented a deep sense of isolation, loneliness, and longing for a sense of belonging in a world in a world that was experienced as a painful, lonely, and profoundly alienating place. A deep sense of alienation from other people could have failed to nourish the existential need for belonging manifesting in visions and creative work. Visions also involved images of outer body experiences and the connection between mind, body, and spirit. Spiritual growth and a sense of the suffering and injustice of the world emerged in the Miami data. Overcoming drug problems was related to spiritual development because spirituality provided participants with meaningful social and spiritual bonds and sense of belonging. Drug use was described as a destructive behavior that only served to enhance and perpetuate emotional separation through escapism. Spiritual development helped participants to control their addiction. Meaning making can manifest itself in visual, symbolic form in spiritual experiences and visions.

Participants discussed visualizing communicative experiences with the HIV virus in their bodies, and this may have reflected attempts to negotiate their HIV by relating to the virus and interacting with it on the level of communication. Some felt that the HIV virus had its own awareness and was a living entity, and visualized HIV as a sentient being with a symbiotic relationship to their bodies. Developing a symbiotic relationship with HIV gave participants a sense of control over their bodies. Regardless of the etiology of these visualizations, the symbolism within these visions was a glimpse into their inner construction of meaning making of HIV and biographical experience. Views of HIV were multidimensional and rooted in life experience and these views of HIV were a critical aspect of trajectories of personal growth. However, negative conceptions of the cause of having HIV can perpetuate negative views of the spiritual and of the self. Therefore, when examining how people living with HIV cope with their illness, spiritual coping and spiritual support seeking processes emerged as an important aspect of their experiences that needed to be considered in the broader context of their lives.

Religious practices themselves were tools utilized for various purposes. Participants reported using religion as a coping mechanism, as a means to repent for sins, and as a weapon to combat stigma. Some participants reported speaking to the church to increase awareness of HIV and used religious institutions as a vehicle and venue for changing public conceptions of illness. Furthermore, making connections between the body, mind, and spirit in relation to health suggest that spirituality and views towards religious institutions were related to health beliefs and behavior. The relationship between spirituality and religion to health behaviors, such as taking medication can be rooted in cultural differences in views of health and illness. This potential connection has implications for health interventions and strategies of implementing medical treatment centers in different cultural contexts. Shared meaning is critical for health initiatives to be effective.

In regards to views of medicine, participants reported a spectrum of views of their physicians ranging from positive and beneficial to negative and inefficient in treatment of HIV. These differences in views of medicine appeared to be rooted in the intersection of social positions and their corresponding biographical experiences. Cultural conceptions of illness and religion and spirituality were related to patients' views of medical treatment and their evaluations of interactions with their doctors and satisfaction with care.

Many participants reported experiencing adverse side effects due to HIV medication. Medication use was also attributed as the cause of friends' deaths due to HIV and taking medication was described as stressful and disrupting homeostasis. The issue of who and what institution was given the power to treat illness by the patients themselves was related to their view of medicine

Also, a preference for holistic treatment was discussed and some participants felt that they were often more knowledgeable about current HIV treatments than their physicians. Using holistic medicine was an alternative that gave participants more control and flexibility in their approaches to their treatment. Problems in continuity of care were discussed in the Miami sample. Experiences of going through multiple doctors before finding the right fit for patients' needs and that they could afford was a problem. Participants in the Miami sample tended to have a series of physicians due to insurance coverage issues, suggesting a problem in continuity of care related to the American health care system. The Ryan White Program was discussed as helping in continuity of care. Similar to the Frankfurt sample, medical treatment served as a reminder of HIV and brought HIV into a daily awareness context. Having to see doctors served as a daily reminder of HIV.

Medication was a double-edged sword. On the one hand, medication helped to transform HIV from a death sentence to a chronic illness. On the other hand, medication often was related to a range of negative side effects. Another negative aspect of taking HIV medication that emerged in both samples was HIV medication as a daily reminder of HIV which brought HIV to the center of awareness and rendered daily life as problematized by HIV status. The high cost of HIV medication and problems with continuity of care due to insurance coverage which often forced people to change their doctors even when they were satisfied with their care was an issue reported in the Miami sample but not in the Frankfurt sample. The institutional context of governmental policy and its role in health care thus shaped the personal experience of HIV treatment. The importance of health care, immigration, and social policy is further discussed on the section on structural conditions of negotiating HIV. Interestingly, process structures of action did not always involve action that benefited the biography incumbent. The emergence of the biographical process of the reversal of agency emerged in the case of Walter and is discussed below.

3.6   Reversal of Agency: Denial and the Construction of Alternate Reality

Walter's denial of HIV can be conceptualized as a reversal of agency. He focused his energy to create an alternative world where he felt he was placed in an experiment against his will. This world was constructed in order to protect him from threat. By remaining in an experiment of his own creation, he was able to maintain his identity as being HIV-negative. Walter displayed a strong desire for control in his life, and this desire for control motivated his construction of HIV as an experiment. Walter was a unique case demonstrating a process where agency was turned against the self. As indicated in the case of Walter, the self has temporal dimensions. Therefore, the self may not know what it will need in the future because the self and life conditions change in unknown and unanticipated ways. Walter was unknowingly in a temporal struggle against his future self because what he perceived as being good for himself at the present had the unintended consequence of entrapping and harming his future self by denying his new identity as HIV-positive.

Because he was in denial of his HIV, Walter did not identify with other people with HIV, seek support, or accept his illness, which in the long-term may have unintended consequences for his health and well-being, preventing him from overcoming a misalignment of his identity or from utilizing resources in the HIV-positive community. Walter was already experiencing some strain due to his maintenance of the experiment construction of HIV which he discussed in regards to the issues of conflicts in "being real" and the need to engage in "ethical persuasion" in order to manage everyday social encounters which are further discussed in the section on disclosure. Walter's agency was turned against himself because of a discrepancy between past and present, or present and future selves. The discrepancy between his conceptions of himself as HIV-negative versus HIV-positive created a temporal divide as he forced HIV out of his awareness and self-concept. His maintenance of his present self was driven by his strong will and desire to maintain control over his identity, driving his rebellion against an HIV-positive identity.

This illustrates an important issue in regards to agency and action. Human agency can have unintended consequences of harming the self when there are incongruities based in struggles of meaning related to self-conceptions and social constructions of categories associated with social positions and statuses, such as HIV. Struggles with meaning can contribute to temporal divisions in identity as the undesired is pushed outside of the present and illusion is maintained. Action can occur through different mechanisms, which can shape self-views and behavior and a reversal of agency can lead to self-destructive behavior. This may explain the difference between Walter and Chris in regards to their approaches towards sexual behavior. Walter was in an internal struggle where he maintained his past self by denying the existence of HIV and in doing so denied any harm that could be done to others through his own actions. Walter's desire to be sexually attractive and to maintain his secret drove his decision to not disclose and to not use condoms.

Chris struggled with the same issues as Walter, but because Chris accepted the reality of HIV and had an open awareness context as he acknowledged his HIV, he practiced safe sex. There were actual consequences for Chris, the harm of another's well-being by HIV transmission, which prevented him from having unprotected sex. The awareness contexts of Walter (closed) versus Chris (open) shaped their sexual behavior (Strauss et al. 1997). Walter was unable to move forward and accept his HIV because he closed HIV out of his awareness and didn't want to be a group member of the HIV-positive community. Walter did not relate to people with HIV, rather he identified himself as an active member of the Hip Hop community and as a musician. His strong prejudice against HIV drove him to close out HIV from his awareness in a very active way. Interestingly, although Walter would write music, he said that his writing was to inform others and not himself. Walter did not talk about HIV in his music because he felt HIV was something he had not yet "grasped" and because of a deep fear of losing his status in the Hip Hop community. Not discussing HIV in his music not only demonstrated his very active closure against the reality of HIV, but also prevented Walter from informing others about HIV with his music, thus preventing any social change.

Acceptance of HIV may have been easier for Chris because he didn't have such strong negative views against HIV, which may be related to his gay collective identity. Initiatives, information, self-help groups, and political movements in the gay community may have been resources that Chris had access to by sharing a collective identity of the gay community. Arthur discussed vast changes in attitudes towards gays in German society. Paragraph 175, a law against homosexual behavior, was in effect when Arthur was younger. However, at the time of the interview, being gay was no longer a crime and Arthur emphasized this as a major positive change. Therefore, the societal change in treatment of gays, such as decriminalization, served to create a more positive environment and tolerance of gays, empowering the gay community and enabling mobilization of resources. In contrast, racism and public attitudes towards African Americans may not have undergone such a positive transformation and Walter may have had to contend with the stress of both racism and HIV. Walter had to deal with HIV, which he defined as out of his control, dirty, and beneath him. In contrast, Arthur was aware that HIV could happen and his diagnosis did not completely alter his view of himself or his social outlook as dramatically as in the case of Walter. The intersection of collective identities can have an important impact on how HIV is experienced. The life experience of a gay white man with HIV can be vastly different than that of a straight black man due to the characteristics associated with each social category and their intersectional meaning.

The identification of the process of agency reversal helps to develop conceptualizations of action because reversal of agency emphasizes how action can be based in identity and time, and can be used against the self unknowingly. Action appeared to be rooted in identity because action was tied to self-conceptions and the desire to act in ways that minimized undesirable aspects of the self and to maximize the valued aspects of self. Furthermore, agency is rooted in time because identity is temporal and is related to the manifestation of action. Walter's closed awareness context and strong prejudice against HIV was a very active form of closure, preventing him from understanding his HIV, relating to others with HIV, and moving forward to deal with this new social reality.

Walter possessed a collective identity based in the world of music and rooted in his ethnicity. African American racial/ethnic identity may not have undergone as much of a shift as being gay in terms of societal acceptance and in regards to information and resources to deal with HIV. Gay political movements have empowered gay communities, and the collective identity of gayness has undergone a dramatic shift. However, despite civil rights movements, racism remains a major issue in contemporary American society (Jones 2000; Blascovich et al. 2001). Exposure to racism may also have increased Walter's strain and difficulty in relating to HIV. Group membership and collective identity can shape resources and attitudes towards HIV, affecting biographical vulnerability dispositions (Betts et al. 2004).

For Walter, HIV presented a stereotype threat and involved a fear of being defined as gay and being stigmatized (Steele and Aronson 1995). Walter did not have a social group he could relate to that he felt would provide mutual acceptance upon his HIV disclosure. Walter explained:

> "Like I said 'You got HIV, oh AIDS that's it you're finished.' Know what I mean? Um like I said I deal with hip hop (-) in the rap world we have somebody/thing called the gay rapper nobody knew who the gay rapper was (-) no one knows there's a gay rapper in hip hop and that's just been going around (-) you know everyone's talking about the gay rapper 'Oh maybe this person's the gay rapper' 'No maybe that person's the gay rapper' but you don't know (-) nobody knows (-) you know what I'm saying? But it was a rumor (-) that's just an example know what I mean? And um whoever that person was or is you hear nothing else about him (-) his career is done (-) whoever he was (-) it's done." [Transcript 1, lines 875-889]

Walter's Hip Hop stance and strong masculine identity worked against him closing his awareness to HIV. Social identity theory supports this analysis with its emphasis on how people: define their selves in relation to the groups they belong to, define themselves in terms of the social and personal, discriminate against groups that pose a threat to group identity, and dissociate from groups that can discredit them and thus group identification can be a response to stigma, either hindering or facilitating action (Howard 2000; Tajfel and Turner 1986). For example, although Walter's mother had HIV, he did not relate to his mother and so he couldn't connect HIV with any self-meaning. In contrast, Rachel's mother helped her to accept HIV, the difference between Walter and Rachel was Rachel's relationship of trust with her mother. This highlights the relational aspect of action where compassionate love and giving and receiving care can facilitate action. This helps to explain the difference between Walter and Rachel and their views on living "double lives." Both Rachel and Walter felt they were living "double lives." Walter was trying to keep spheres of music and HIV separate, the separation of social worlds can be both productive and counterproductive. The difference in the outcome of the maintenance of separation of social worlds was acceptance of HIV and the creation of meaningful connections between different worlds.

The world of music and entertainment was essential to Walter's conception of reality and world view. Conceptions of knowledge and truth emerged clearly in the cases of Walter and Chris who both were recently diagnosed one year ago at the time of their interviews. Reflective debates about the nature of reality may indicate the existential struggle that these newly diagnosed men faced in making sense of reality and attempting to regain a sense of coherence, which is an important aspect of biographical work. Walter placed a great deal of emphasis on fantasy and illusion and the role of entertainment and government in obscuring the true nature of reality. Walter believed that information was placed in entertainment (in movies, music, and writing) and must be found in order for people to be free. He explained:

> "You watch the (-) you watch movies Harry Potter (-) uh harr (-) uh Lord of the Rings these are signs but we not really looking you know (voice raises to questioning tone) we (-) we (-) we're not looking but these are signs (-) just look (-) open your eyes up (-) don't just be entertained it's not just about entertainment." [Transcript 1, lines 1053-1063]

Walter used movies as an example. Specifically, he chose popular movies to demonstrate that entertainment and the content of cinema were not to be interpreted at a superficial level. Rather, he felt there were "signs" which were overlooked in entertainment which we must open our eyes to see. He argued that the purpose of entertainment was not just to "entertain" or amuse an audience, there existed a truth to be found. Walter worked in the entertainment industry as a musician and this may be why entertainment was an important part of his awareness context. Also, he provided his conception of truth:

> "A wise man told me you can't really have a lie without some type of truth (-) you know a lie can't exist without some type of truth it doesn't have to be full truth (-) you know what I mean? It's gotta be some type of truth for that lie to exist" [Transcript 1; lines 1065-1071]

Was entertainment then a lie? Was fiction nonfiction? Was this what he meant by saying that "a lie can't exist without some type of truth"? Was this why Walter chose popular movies, which were both based on fiction novels, specifically in the genre of fantasy, to discuss entertainment? For Walter, the truth and lies could not exist without each other. What was known was uncertain. The distinction between truth and lies was softened, what was known contained both truth and lies. If this is how he perceived the world, then how could anything truly ever be known? What was the truth? He further explained:

> "Don't look on the surface (-) kinda look underneath don't just look at 'Entertainment's entertainment' (-) cause a lot of stuff it isn't just entertainment there's a lot of information out there for us to see if you're not aware (-) just walk around dumb (-) blindfolded and no problem" [Transcript 1; lines 1073-1079].

Entertainment was portrayed as based on illusion and fantasy, as being a lie which within it held a truth. According to Walter, that truth was found in information within entertainment. Walter felt that entertainment was a medium to increase knowledge if one thinks critically and does not accept it at face value. Because Walter felt that there were people who live their lives unaware of the truth to be found in their surroundings, and that people accept things at face value, he separated himself and identified himself as knowledgeable, active, and aware. If people are ignorant this allowed the potential for others to have power over them by their possession of privileged knowledge. Walter sought control over his life and so he searched for knowledge. The pursuit of truth held great meaning to Walter. Therefore, Walter's reversal of agency was tied to not only his identity, but to his view of the world, knowledge, and the truth. By refusing to accept HIV and insisting on an alternate and hidden reality, as expressed by his beliefs in conspiracy theory and suspicion of authority, Walter's agency was unwittingly turned against the needs of his new self with HIV. HIV was related to Walter's search for the truth as he emphasized:

> "I tell the people (-) I tell you the things I tell you the things that I say this is why with my music (-) you know what I'm saying (-) I just try to (--) 'Look another way' know what I'm saying? Don't just look for the surface (-) look underneath (-) and it's the same shit I'm dealing with this HIV shit (taps loudly) it's a little deeper than me just having this, or this just coming to me, 'How did this come to me?' ok if it is (-) 'Where?' 'How?' 'Why?' You know? And my only question is, in this whole HIV thing, is why is not this chick that I've been with for three years (-) with no knowledge (-) no awareness of me having this (-) not infected?" [Transcript 1, lines 1106-1115]

Walter felt that the truth involved more than him being told he had HIV and he wanted answers. He had a need to understand the etiology of HIV, the processes involved, and the meaning or purpose of HIV. Walter needed answers to these questions in order for him to accept that he had HIV, and approached the media and conceptions of commonly accepted truths in a parallel style of understanding and meaning making. Therefore, what he debated in the media symbolized what he considered important to daily life and what he conceived of as problematic in his experiences. This also suggests that cultural symbols embedded in the media are not passively received but instead can be negotiated into existing schemes of meaning. Negotiations of new images with existing knowledge can be a negotiation which is private and representative of otherwise invisible processes in the formulation of meaning and of resolving internal dilemmas between the self and experience.

Walter did not relate to others with HIV, he did not have a social reference group to relate to, so he covered his stigma completely and hid his identity as someone with HIV. He was even closed off to himself, if he does not eventually come to terms with HIV as being real, he may develop a negative view of his treatment and medication and have problems with adherence to treatment. For now, he took his medication "just in case" but he already was developing a distrust of medicine as perhaps even maintaining HIV in his body. Therefore, Walter may have been on the verge of acceptance that he kept at bay by pushing the potential realness of HIV away from his awareness context. Perhaps Walters felt that accepting treatment was accepting the care of others and admitting vulnerability, and so he associated care with being passive and vulnerable, which contradicted his view of himself as autonomous and strong. This suspicion of care closed off a major source of support and empowerment to Walter. Medical care and economic resources can be seen as instrumental to regaining a sense of control over life after HIV diagnosis. Participants emphasized financial resources and support in medical care as discussed below.

3.7   Financial Freedom and Autonomy:
The Importance of Economic Resources in Regaining Autonomy

Importantly, the biographical effects of economic resources on dealing with HIV were emphasized. Action was also facilitated by processes emergent on the structural level of economic opportunity and of access to financial resources. For example, Arthur defined work as a means of achieving autonomy and financial freedom and explained:

> "I was kind of lucky that I was able to retire at a very early age (-) at the same amount of money I was working (-) I had a good job like I said (-) I made some quite good money and then didn't need to go to work and start a second life actually with the infection (-) I was lucky (-) I had bad luck when I caught the infection (-) but on the other hand I was lucky with the treatment medical (-) medical wise and didn't need to go to work again (-) so I had another start (-) a second life." [Transcript 4, lines 29-35]

This transition out of work was a turning point in his life because this is where Arthur began a "second life" and no longer had to work. Arthur made a distinction between "good" and "bad" luck as he described his life situation. Financial freedom was emphasized and allowed Arthur to be free of the occupational sphere of work. The world of work for Arthur was an interesting place because, on the one hand, he was successful in his profession, but yet on the other hand he was not free because he had to keep the secret of being both gay and having HIV in this sphere of his life. Financial freedom allowed him to be free from his "closeted life" and to start anew. Financial freedom was a key factor in his biographical process of regaining autonomy and taking action. Notably, he felt that such financial freedom would likely not occur in the American system:

> "I was able to go on disability that's how you call it over here and uh if you get it over here you get your regular pension more or less (-) In America that's different (-)and uh so I didn't have any problems like financially and I got the medication from here (-) the medication is free here too (-) the health system over here is much more uh for the people I should say (-) not so much for like the Americans the HMO things (-) Kaiser (-) Permante[3] all that shit I experienced (-) I had an American friend over there and on occasion to deal with them too (-) so here you don't need to worry if you had a job before (-) paid your social security things in so you get your pension and retirement money and so you don't need to worry actually (-) America that's different." [Transcript 4, lines 128-137]

Arthur explained that the German system was different than the American system, and because of the policies of the German system, he did not experience any financial stress. Not only did the German system allow him to receive his pension, but it also provided him with free medication. Arthur felt that the German health care system, as compared to the American system was "much more for the people." Arthur brought up these international comparisons of health care without any prompting. David also compared the American and German healthcare systems and strongly believed that the financial support of German health insurance in paying for HIV medication was a major factor that allowed people with HIV to survive and to avoid falling into poverty.

Structural conditions such as health care policy, which shape access to resources, can be facilitating conditions affecting action on the structural level. Without economic and medical resources, action could not be taken in order to maintain positive health behaviors such as medication adherence and treatment of HIV. David emphasized the critical role that the German health insurance system played in patient's care and felt that without the support of the insurance system and its financing of HIV medication, his quality of life would be severely limited and that other patients who were in more vulnerable positions than himself would die without the resources provided by the German health care

---

3   Kaiser Permante is an organization which provides HIV health care services in the United States.

system. Medication access and affordability, financial stability, and social security were seen as critical to the maintenance of health and survival.

Access to material resources through informal networks was also discussed by participants in Miami. Perceived instrumental support refers to the belief that significant others are available to provide financial or other forms of tangible assistance such as transportation, housing, or even caregiving. Some participants discussed having someone they can rely on to borrow money from in times of need or someone who can or has provided assistance such as borrowing a car, giving them rides to work or to run errands. Social support can come from family, friends, intimate partners, doctors, and the community. In a context of socioeconomic disadvantage, instrumental social support can be especially important. Economic hardship and financial problems were pronounced among the Miami sample. Participants emphasized the importance of instrumental support, such as assistance with transportation, neighbors sharing food, and governmental support in medical care and financial support. In the context of perpetual poverty, some participants in Miami even felt that having HIV had provided them with more support from the government because it allowed them to meet the eligibility requirements for governmental assistance. Participants in Miami reflected on the need for the American welfare and health care systems to be improved in order to provide support for people suffering from deeply rooted inequality. There was a perceived need to remove the disability requirements for governmental support. This suggests that the removal of a disability requirement for support in more recent governmental legislation has been an improvement to the previous policies surrounding health care.

Participants in Miami felt it was a problem that to get assistance from the government they were required to have HIV and felt that the welfare system needed to be improved. Descriptions of not being able to afford enough food or to qualify for Medicaid were recurrent themes in the Miami interviews. In order to be eligible for Medicaid, participants' incomes in Miami had to remain at a very low level. The low-income requirements of Medicaid could contribute to a perpetuation of poverty by preventing people who need assistance in medical care from working to achieve higher incomes.

An important distinction between the Miami and Frankfurt samples was that in Germany, participants felt that the support they received from the government fit their needs and allowed them to obtain quality medical care and to afford their medication. Participants in Germany even wondered how people in the United States survive and deal with HIV in a context of a more limited social security system, and felt that many people would die without the support they were receiving. In Germany, participants were able to obtain medical coverage and support without having to stop their careers in order to go on disability. Because having a professional career was important to participants, this suggests that such policy requirements to meet eligibility for medical coverage in the United States can limit professional and personal development of people with HIV. While not generalizable, it is notable that the Miami sample tended to be economically disadvantaged whereas the Frankfurt sample did not report poverty.

Medicine was described as poison, and HIV was felt as an ongoing battle in the Miami sample, and this was similar to the case of Walter who had a negative view of medicine and used violent metaphors when describing HIV. Because of the wealth of the U.S., it is unlikely that other nations will contribute to programs to assist people living in poverty with HIV in the U.S. However, because of the deeply rooted and vast inequality in income in the U.S., which serves to perpetuate cumulative advantages and disadvantages and an unequal distribution of resources, it is unlikely that the American elite would support funding and structural changes that would fundamentally alter the distribution of resources. The individualistic culture of the United States, which can be traced to the Protestant ethic and capitalism, locates the source of social problems within the individual, thus diverting attention away from structural problems (Weber 1930).

Economic inequality could be further problematized by antagonistic race relations. Witnessing racial violence and was described in tandem with a desire to humanity to bring unity and to end suffering. The intersection of racism and economic inequality can create a context of isolation and powerlessness. In the absence of meaningful and compassionate bonds with people which cross racial and economic boundaries, inequality and separation can continue to serve as major barriers to overcoming health disparities in HIV. As discussed by participants, poverty and social inequality is a major concern in contemporary American society, which is particularly troubling in the case of HIV where simple, taken for granted aspects of daily life can be problematized by poverty and by illness. Practical daily concerns appeared to affect health behaviors. Having financial support was important to participants and concerns regarding the American health care and welfare as inefficient system of support for people in need were expressed in the Miami sample. Poverty was a persistent problem in a context of perpetual economic disadvantage and lack of governmental support.

The importance of instrumental support as a resource was pronounced in the Miami sample where more participants reported financial hardship, restricted employment, and neighborhood disadvantage. The problem of perpetual economic disadvantage was also continuously expressed by those with high levels of educational attainment and prestigious careers who expressed concerns over their finances. Resources were described as being so limited that they affected participants' ability to properly care for their health. Participants in Miami had to adapt the best way they could in the context of limited financial resources. Financial stress was a common concern among the Miami sample, even when participants had high levels of education attainment and prior professional careers. In a context of socioeconomic disadvantage, an important aspect of HIV patients' lives was the reality of illness among their loved ones in their lives and financial problems in paying for their medical care.

Economic concerns played important roles in participants' lives and decisions. A troubling concern were the descriptions of having to not accept employment offers because if they had an income that surpassed a threshold they would no longer have access to financial support in order to receive their medication and health care.

An important issue for people living with HIV in America was medical coverage for HIV medication and treatment. In order to be able to afford treatment, most participants had to receive Medicaid and to no longer be employed full-time and to have low-incomes. This was a major issue because employment can allow an improved standard of living, a fulfilling career, structured daily life, and opportunities for interaction in a professional setting. Because of this limitation in the American health care system, many participants were not allowed a viable opportunity to develop professionally in an occupational setting. Some participants responded to this restriction by being involved in a number of entrepreneurial and creative projects. Economic resources were needed to launch creative projects participants discussed how they had to work to make money to fund their creative and self-directed work in the context of limited resources. The biographical processes identified here thus appeared to overlap.

3.8   Action Process Structures: Additional Comments

As demonstrated in the above cases, biographical process structures were embedded in life experience, social context, resources, and personal and cultural biographies. The action process structures that were identified in this analysis occurred at different levels of social reality and should not be considered as exhaustive, but rather as conceptualizations of biographical experience which can overlap and intersect with one another to affect the realization and utilization of agency. It is possible that action can manifest itself in many more ways and at more levels of social reality.

Therefore, while the analysis of these cases helped me to identify biographical process structures of action, other processes were identified in the supplemental cases analyzed and these processes demonstrated overlap. For example, Nancy's experience in giving birth was important in her taking action and compassionate love along with support seeking via participation in Helping Hand empowered her. In addition, financial freedom along with participation in Helping Hand was reported as extremely helpful and empowering to David. Giving compassionate love to children and engaging in extensive biographical work through her psychoanalysis empowered Sarah to remain active and to maintain her career and the well-being of her family. Multiple processes can be involved in biographical development and action and while conceptually distinct they appeared to share overlap in biographical experience. Negotiation of HIV involved the realization of agency and the engagement in action. The intersection of internal, relational, and structural aspects of biographical experience appeared to be important to participants' action schemes. Empowerment can be conceived of as the regaining of control over adverse life circumstances and a sense of power, strength, and deep meaning, which was deeply intertwined with the enactment of agency and motivated people to improve their lives and the lives of others.

Another action process structure emerged in the case of George. Closeness with death empowered George, attuned him to his personal strength, and helped him to find more value and meaning in life. Interestingly, prior research has found that near-death experiences can serve as turning points among people with HIV (Kremer et al. 2009). George described two near-death experiences. The first was a drastic weight loss which occurred when he was as a young gay man struggling with anorexia. George's anorexia lead him to lose fifty kilograms in one year and he was extremely ill. George reported that this experience prepared him to face his next near-death experience when he was seriously ill due to HIV. George was misdiagnosed with cancer and had a drastic drop in his white blood cells and felt close to death. George's familiarity and acceptance of death helped him to cope with his HIV. Action appeared to manifest itself at the biographical level of personal growth and strength in the face of death. Thus, there can be many ways on different levels of social reality through which agency is realized and conceptualizing agency as process-based and intimately tied with action, and occurring in different levels of social reality, could further develop the concept of agency.

3.9   Part 3: Theoretical Aspects of Negotiating HIV

Thus far, the emergent themes in the overarching aspects of conditions for the emergence of trajectory of suffering and of various biographical processes involved in living with HIV have been discussed. Here, the theoretical aspects of negotiating HIV are examined. These aspects emerged in both the Frankfurt and Miami samples and appear to be fundamental aspects of living with HIV. Disclosure and stigma both were intimately related aspects of negotiating HIV and are discussed below.

3.9.1   Disclosure and Living with HIV as a Secret

Strauss (1997) maintained that human interaction is fraught with danger because our social relationships are fluid and subject to change. The inherent danger in interaction is especially prominent for PLWHA because of the stigmatized nature of the social meaning ascribed to HIV. HIV disclosure holds the risk of a complete restructuring of social relationships and devastating social losses. Therefore, examining the inherent danger of HIV disclosure may also provide an opportunity to examine the normalization and maintenance of social relationships because these aspects of social life are especially pronounced for PLWHA. Others without HIV may engage in similar types of processes when deciding on what information to reveal to others and when deciding on their mode of presentation of self. Considerations of others' reactions to new information related to one's identity or social status can shape how people choose to present themselves to the world. This corresponds to identity control theory (ICT) which focuses on the meaning-based nature of identity rooted in social structural arrangements and processes of information control in negotiating identity in social interaction (Burke 2007; 1991).

The world manifest due to these presentations of self can be substantially different than the hidden world of identities not revealed to others. For example, Chris was a gay teacher with HIV and Sarah was the mother of two young boys in school. Both Chris and Sarah feared to disclose to others at their schools. However, what was the true nature of their respective school settings? Secrets render social settings as having potential for a division between external and internal reality. Nothing may be as it appeared. A social setting can be seen as a social grouping of people who all have their own modes of presentation of self that shape each person's action and reaction to another. What would happen if

Sarah's children had had Chris as their kindergarten teacher? What would happen if both disclosed their HIV status to one another? Yet it is likely that this possibility would not be allowed by both parties. No participants reported being completely open and out about their HIV status in the Frankfurt sample. HIV disclosure was a serious decision and participants disclosed very selectively. Many participants discussed that their HIV was a "secret" that they had to carry and some participants conceptualized living the secret of HIV as living a "double life." Accordingly, Chris described an awareness of the inherent danger that the admission of his HIV status could have. Chris observed others discussing HIV and provided an example:

> "I catch myself feeling like 'Wow ok um this is really awkward this feels like really weird but no one knows' like for example I went to a party like a month ago and uh um we all had drinks and they all had these red cups so we drank and no one knew which cup was whose and they were like one of the friends she was like 'it's not like we have AIDS you know just drink out of one' and I was like 'Wow I could have totally I could have been like that a year ago not knowing that I'm positive' being like 'Ok I'm just gonna joke about it' but (-) cause they're not trying to be hurtful or anything but it's just like a joke I'm like a joke that people like to make like 'Oh yeah you can give me a kiss it's not like (--) or you can drink out of my cup it's not like I have AIDS or stuff' so that tells me um just by saying that people really do think if you drink out of the same cup you could get it you know?" [Transcript 3, lines 160-171]

An awareness of stigma and an observation of negative attitudes towards HIV without revealing his HIV status rendered this situation as "awkward" and "weird." Chris observed this casual joke about HIV and felt that he could have said something similar a year ago before he was HIV-positive. Chris did not feel that people who speak about HIV were deliberately trying to be hurtful; rather he viewed them as joking when they made offhanded and uninformed references about HIV/AIDS. However, jokes and comments signified to Chris that people were ignorant of HIV as he elaborated:

> "They use the word AIDS but HIV and AIDS are like two different things you know (-) like HIV is just you know a disease and AIDS (-) if it like breaks out (-) if it's like towards the end I'll say now (--) so that tells me or shows me that people really don't know anything about it it's used um everyone knows it's there but "Ok as long as I'm not affected by it (-) I'm just not gonna think about it or I'll just try to avoid it." [Transcript 3, lines 173-178]

Entry into the HIV-positive community allowed access to information which was not previously in one's stock of knowledge as Chris told:

"I'm not saying I'm glad I have it but it's **I'm glad** that I have the knowledge now because if it wouldn't have happened to me um who knows? I'd be one of those ignorant people running around judging (-) pointing you know and just that's the good thing that came out of it (-) like I have more knowledge (-) I'm more understanding then I was before and um yeah (-) I think now I'm able to help people in that situation by um telling them my story or it's even good that I'm here now you know that I can do something good with it it's yeah (-) it's one of the good parts (-)." [Transcript 3, lines 297-302]

HIV remained a secret for those interviewed that was carefully handled. The world of secrets does not belong to the working world where people can act to change the external. The world of secrets can be considered a part of the realm of phantasms as conceptualized by Alfred Schütz (Schütz 1962) which is similar to the world of dreams. The world of secrets can be considered a world of waking dreams which has two fundamental implications: 1. One remains alone in both dreams and in secrets and is thus solely responsible for the maintenance of secrecy and isolated from others 2. One cannot change the working world because the secret remains outside the realm of actualization and human action and thus cannot alter social relationships or external reality. This highlights the emphasis placed on keeping HIV a secret. Secrecy served to protect from social losses and to maintain the normalcy of social relationships. However, by remaining in the world of secrets, the bearer of the secret of HIV lost the power to fundamentally challenge the conceptions and negative attitudes surrounding HIV in the working world. The secret of HIV highlights the hidden aspects of managed identities which play a subtle role in interaction. The issues of illusion and truth and the divide between the external and the inner or true nature of the self and social relationships were pronounced in the case of HIV. For example, Sarah discussed her decision to not disclose to people in her small town in Germany:

"Not in (-) not in our city anyway (-) because I live in a small town and there is much gossip going around (-) you know people everyone knows everyone and uh you know these things are difficult (-) the social control is very tight and uh so they still don't know anything." [Transcript 5, lines 72-78]

The social conditions of her everyday life living in a small town shaped Sarah's attitude towards HIV disclosure. She felt that in the small town where she lived there was a lack of anonymity, "everyone knows everyone," gossip was prevalent, and the "social control is very tight." Sarah was aware of the closeness of the social networks in her community and their ability to spread information in an identifiable way. She felt that these social networks therefore were constraining and constituted a form of "social control" over her behavior and how she had to manage her presentation of self. To admit her HIV status to even one person in this social context was fraught with danger due to the easy diffusion of this information to others. Therefore, Sarah maintained this secret in order to protect herself from gossip and to maintain a socially desirable presentation of self. Presentation of self was important in how Sarah behaved and felt towards others. A keen awareness of visibility, social networks, and a feeling of being socially controlled were all factors shaping her mode of presentation of self as HIV-negative.

Because HIV was a secretive aspect of her identity this highlighted the importance of Erving Goffman's (Goffman 1959) formulation of presentation of self in daily life and its implications for social interaction and identity. Sarah's mode of presentation of self as being HIV-negative created a divide between her inner identity as HIV-positive and the manifest presentation she showed to the world. The divide between this major aspect of her identity and what she felt that she must show to the world created a burden. Being unable to disclose for Sarah appeared to mean a separation of her inner and outer identities, which divided and burdened her emotionally. Similarly, Walter and Rachel used the term of living a "double life." Rachel explained:

> "(Exhales) I don't know(-) I still have this feeling it's not as strong as before but it's (--) now now I (-) it's like I'm living a double life (-) when I have you as my friend we (-) we go (-) we live this other way and then when I am (-) when I am here with the people who are positive that is another life too (-) so yeah (-) I separate this (-) both lives for me it's different (laughs nervously) they are two different lives (-) positive or not being positive (-) so when I'm in a community where people are negative I live like a negative person and when I'm here (-) I'm living another way (-) and so I can talk the people here (-) the ways about the sickness (-) and if someone ask you know 'yeah'." [Transcript 2, lines 330-342]

Rachel lived two different lives, in one life she lived as an HIV-positive person and in her other life she lived "like a negative person." When Rachel was in the HIV-positive community, she felt she could talk about HIV and be open. Living a double life allowed Rachel to keep her secret of HIV from those she felt couldn't under-stand her, but also allowed her to speak about HIV freely with people who were part of the HIV-positive community. Rachel was flexible and able to adapt by switching between the HIV-positive and HIV-negative worlds and acting or living as other members of each world in order to blend in. Rachel therefore managed her presentation of self-consciously and purposely. Rachel's ability to do this enabled her to cope with her HIV status, to maintain her privacy in the HIV-negative world, and to prevent violations of trust or the potential de-legitimatization of her identity while still maintaining her identity as being HIV-positive but in a supportive and safe environment. HIV was a secret she carried and secrets require continuous maintenance in order to not be discovered in everyday life. Similarly, Walter told:

> "Now (-) see that (-) now see that's (-) see that's this is a secret that I have to bear with (-) I have to live with I can't tell this (3) you know I can't be free about this "hey listen what's happening man? What's going on? I got HIV. Let's go drink one." You know what I'm saying? "Let's sit down and have a cigarette I have HIV, you know let's just chill out" (-) you know you just can't do that you know so now (-) now you're kinda living a (-) by me knowing this this kinda threw me into a Clark Kent Superman so to speak (-) identity (-) you know what I mean? At one point (-) you know, in one sense I'm "yeah you know" I'm that "hey what's happening people?" people know me in this sense but then, there's a dark (--) I'm keeping a secret that I can't (---) let out (-) know what I'm saying? That door cannot be opened." [Transcript 1, lines 435-446]

Walter's knowledge of his HIV status was a special type of knowledge, it was privatized, and not to be shared. Secrets have implications for expressions of self and relations to others. Walter's freedom was restricted by his knowledge that within him was this virus, and without him were those who could not, or would not understand his reality. Walter depicted the image of a potential scenario in everyday life and how it would be altered by his disclosure of having HIV "Hey listen what's happening man? What's going on? I got HIV. Let's go drink one." A normal social interaction would be irrevocably altered by Walter's admission of his HIV status. Walter felt this would be socially unacceptable because doing so would alter other's conceptions of Walter and his social encounters with others. So Walter told no one. He did not want to carry the consequences of being labeled as having HIV; instead he chose to bear the burden of his secret alone. This suggests that secrets can constitute a form of privatized and privileged knowledge, which hurt and can yet empower us. The secret of HIV was described as "heavy" and "a burden" as David explained:

> "It is always heavy this secret, this is heavy because you always think 'They might find out' you're very careful to speak about things." (Sequential Report 8, p. 3)

The burden of maintaining the secret of HIV appeared to involve issues of employing modes of presentation of self as HIV-negative in order to create the illusion of being HIV-negative. This highlighted HIV as a social role with strain. This view is consistent with theoretical suggestions regarding the relation of social structure to social roles and strain (Merton 1938; 1957). Researchers have emphasized that stressful life events can be seen as a process where stressful life events can lead to ongoing role strains, which can then impair self-concepts, which then leads to more stress (Pearlin et al. 1981). Role strain has been defined as involving difficulties in fulfilling role demands (Goode 1960). Role strain in the social role of HIV involved the constant maintenance of secrecy, and required a great deal of invisible and emotional work geared at the separation of HIV-positive and HIV-negative spheres of life. For instance, Nancy managed this information with her children by making her taking of medication into a game and other HIV-positive mothers also reported keeping their HIV a secret from their children. This work was reported as stressful and even as denying important aspects of the self as Walter described:

> "I'm a real person (-) like (-) I'm (-) I like dealing with reality, being real, I say what this (-) is what it is (-) this is how it is, that's it (-) by me not being able to say certain things and have to probably beat around the bush or sorta go around so that I wouldn't be forced to be put in that situation where I will have to say something you know what I'm saying? Then it's a lot I'm (1) I'm kinda living a lie." [Transcript 1, lines 448-455]

Walter's avoidance of revealing his HIV status but at the same time avoiding this truth affected his own authenticity and view of himself as being "real." Living a double life, while it allowed Walter to maintain his reputation, made him feel that he was "living a lie" An important issue is why Walter viewed himself as taking on a "superman identity" and carrying a dark secret, whereas Rachel viewed herself as being a member of two communities. One potential reason is that Rachel was a member of an actual HIV-positive community, Helping Hand, whereas Walter did not have membership in an HIV-positive community. Walter was not a member of Helping Hand and felt that he was "in a different class" than the other patients in the clinic. Walter's reference group or community was the Hip Hop community, not the HIV-positive community and he strongly identified himself as a musician. Participants who reported an active and positive identification with the HIV-positive community all reported being members of Helping Hand.

Therefore, HIV was a secret which could be a burden but this secret at the same time allowed for access to specialized and privileged knowledge. The bearers of such knowledge must carry this information in secrecy and transverse efficiently between two worlds. Rachel and Walter negotiated the HIV-positive and HIV-negative worlds by living a double life and other participants selectively disclosed. The stigma of HIV appeared to be instrumental in shaping participant's decisions to keep their HIV as a secret. Participant's comparisons of

HIV to cancer as being an illness which even with a better prognosis could not be discussed with other people due to the view of HIV as being tied to deviant sexual behavior and thus as deeply discrediting demonstrated that stigma and its accompanying potential social losses upon disclosure were major driving forces in participants' life experiences with HIV.

Participants made comparisons of HIV to cancer. George, described HIV as being favorable to cancer. The summer before our interview, George was close to death, hospitalized, and misdiagnosed with cancer. George framed his treatment in the hospital in a very inhumane and degrading manner as he described how physicians removed his bone marrow in front of other patients as he laid on the floor of an open hospital room. George's negative treatment in the hospital and his near-death experience may have shaped his conception of HIV as more favorable.

George described his near-death experience as he was in an ambulance and then in the hospital where he realized he was still alive. He was lying in the emergency part of the hospital and there was an older man next to him and this man was pulling the IV's out of his arm and bleeding onto George's bed. The man was not clean, he defecated in his pants and went to George's bed and his waste was all over his bed. George explained how the staff would keep coming to him with a different diagnosis and after five days, the first person said he had HIV. Therefore, George's HIV diagnosis almost came as a relief because he was deathly ill and thought that he was dying of cancer. The conceptions that George created through his illness experience of cancer appeared to be negative and associated with death and medical mistreatment and this may be why HIV was framed in a favorable light to cancer.

Nancy, who did not report any diagnosis of cancer, also made a favorable comparison of HIV to cancer as she explained how her mother used to counsel people with HIV and how her mother would tell her that she couldn't die, that HIV was not like cancer and as long as she took medication and lived a healthy lifestyle she wouldn't die. Nancy heard this first from her mother before she heard it from the doctors and so she did not feel that HIV was a death sentence. Even though participants viewed cancer as being more fatal than HIV, they were faced with the discrepancy that people without HIV considered HIV to be deadly and socially unacceptable. However, due to a fear of rejection and anticipation of stigma, many participants did not report trying to alter public conceptions of HIV. David was active in discussing HIV in communities and attempted to spread information and awareness about HIV. Despite David's efforts at educating others about HIV, he felt that his efforts were not successful and he even suffered the negative consequence of having his HIV status revealed against his will due to his efforts to educate others. This highlights the issue of HIV as a secret to protect social status and the risk involved in being associated with HIV to reputation. Importantly, participants reported holding similar stereotypes of HIV prior to their own diagnoses, which supports the proposition of modified labeling theory (MLT) (Link et al. 1989) that prior conceptions of social groups shape people's experiences and self-views once they themselves enter the social group in question.

An HIV diagnosis can alter perceptions of others with HIV and grant PLWHA with a privatized and privileged knowledge of HIV. Similar to Chris, Walter's conceptions of HIV were also challenged by his own diagnosis. Walter's diagnosis redefined the way he perceived people with HIV and the causes of HIV group membership. HIV could happen to "normal" people in accidental ways that were not their fault. The example in the form of a metaphor of being in the woods and accidently being cut and having this result in HIV infection was brought in to illustrate the plausibility of accidental causes for HIV infection. Walter's entry into the group of people with HIV began to expand his understanding of HIV infection as being outside the realm of blame. Other interviewees reported an awareness of public conceptions of HIV, which linked HIV to negative stereotypes.

Similar to Walter, Sarah appeared to internalize these stereotypes and felt that she was not a "typical" case of someone with HIV and assumed that her deceased husband engaged in homosexual sex, thus giving her HIV. Chris listened to other's misconceptions but did not tell if he ever attempted to rectify them or how he dealt emotionally with feeling that others were ignorant and rejecting of people with HIV. Chris appeared to cope with this knowledge by justifying other's lack of information by comparing others to his past self and his own conceptions before his HIV diagnosis. Internally, Walter rebelled against HIV. Walter dealt with the management of this secret in social interaction in a unique way that he called "ethical persuasion."

Disclosure was also emphasized by the Miami participants. Interviewees in Miami described disclosure of their HIV status as stressful. Stress related to disclosure can be troublesome. For example, perceived stress of disclosure can decrease the likelihood of HIV disclosure (Kalichman and Simbayi 2003). Many participants reported disclosure-related stress and the potential and experienced impact of disclosure on social relationships was an important concern. Furthermore, some reported that disclosure was stressful due to other's reactions but that it was more stressful to not disclose. Disclosure appeared to be less of an issue for some participants who had lived longer with HIV and became more comfortable with their HIV status. HIV disclosure can be stressful, but as HIV is lived with over time, disclosure can become less stressful. Participants in Miami often disclosed to a small number (approximately 0-3) of close friends, family members, or to their partners.

A diagnosis of HIV can lead to difficulties in social relationships due to loved ones and potential intimate partners withdrawing. Participants in both samples struggled with feelings of rejection. Also similar to the Frankfurt sample, participants in Miami emphasized the importance of physical appearance in how others treated them. Being rejected was devastating and presented an even deeper problem beyond the immediate rejection. Rejection became a new problem in navigating social interaction that was not such an issue prior to diagnosis. Both samples placed a great deal of importance on their popularity, social status, and likeability and how these aspects of their identity were threatened by their HIV status. Participants reported both positive and supportive reactions to HIV disclosure and also negative rejecting reactions. Also similar to Frankfurt participants, Miami participants relayed experiences of rejection due to their disclosure, and disclosure was described as a factor in establishing and maintaining intimate relationships. Reactions of others to HIV disclosure were important in shaping life experiences. Disclosure posed a risk of losing loved ones and intimate partners. Adjusting to separations from intimate partners was stressful and establishing new relationships was difficult with HIV as a concern.

The relationships of care between participants and their children were emphasized in both samples. However, both in Frankfurt and Miami, participants also reported finding love after HIV and finding partners who supported and accepted them despite their HIV. Having supportive relationships appeared to have benefits extending beyond the immediate context of one social relationship and to enhance other relationships. By relating openly and having a fulfilling relationship with intimate partners, some participants were able to and to mend their relationships with their families. Receiving love and acceptance in a relationship can extend to other social relationships, improving life circumstances.

The search for love was difficult. Love was an important driving force for participants. The pursuit of beauty and pleasure emerged in the narratives and highlighted the importance of love in life. The troubles in finding a partner were difficult. Accordingly, many participants expressed the feeling that one of the more stressful aspects of their HIV was disclosing to potential partners and scaring them away. Some preferred to have a partner who also was HIV-positive so that the relationship would be easier to negotiate without fear of infecting their partners. Having an HIV-positive partner sometimes allowed for a shared understanding of each other's life situation. The issue of pregnancy after HIV diagnosis as an "ethical" dilemma and feeling dismissed by physicians when inquiring how to have a safe pregnancy and HIV-negative child emerged in the Miami sample. Age appeared to intersect with HIV status in regards to the negative response upon inquiries about how to have a safe pregnancy.

Disclosure was also selective, some participants disclosed to some family members but not others, to friends but not family, to partners but not others, and some even to employers. In contrast to the Frankfurt sample, some of the Miami participants reported disclosing in the workplace. No participants reported HIV disclosure in the workplace among the Frankfurt sample. In contrast, some participants in Miami described being open about their status in the workplace. Other participants reported eventually becoming open with the HIV status, which allowed them to take action to spread awareness of HIV and to improve the welfare of others.

However, the decision to not disclose HIV status could prevent a more effective approach to reducing HIV stigma as prior research suggests that HIV interventions to increase awareness and to reduce stigma are more effective when the speaker disclosed their HIV status (Scollay et al. 1992). The decision to not disclose can also affect the person not disclosing themselves by perpetuating a life of secrecy, shame, and fear. Secondary stigma or the proliferation of stigma to loved ones was described as a factor limiting disclosure activities and HIV activism. Importantly, after years of trying to increase awareness of HIV some participants withdrew and decided to no longer be open about their status.

In contrast, while participants in the Frankfurt sample reported helping others and being involved in Helping Hand, no participants reported being completely open with their HIV status in Frankfurt. Another difference between the Frankfurt and Miami samples was that the discussion of living a "double life" was not as pronounced in the Miami sample. This may have been due to less openness with HIV disclosure among the Frankfurt sample, which made living a double life more of a salient concern than among the Miami participants who tended to be more open about their HIV status. Participants in both Miami and Frankfurt reported fears of losing their social status, jeopardizing their careers and reputation, and losing people upon disclosure. Both samples had the same fears of rejection and stigma and yet no one in the Frankfurt sample reported being completely open about their HIV status. It is unclear what accounts for this difference. Length of time since diagnosis, while important, was not the defining factor as those living with HIV for long periods of time were interviewed in both samples. Perhaps the cultural climate of the U.S., which emphasizes free speech and especially the openness and cultural diversity in Miami, may have been socio-cultural factors that contributed to being open about HIV. The strong corporate culture and emphasis on maintaining reputation and social credibility in Frankfurt where the sample was interviewed may have hindered openness of HIV. Also, Miami is a city characterized by sexual freedom, a larger population, loss of inhibition, cultural diversity, and sexuality. Miami is not only diverse but has a sizable gay community and this may have helped gay participants to feel more safe in disclosing because there was a sense of gay pride and a gay community to turn to for support and which also was an active entity in raising awareness of HIV in the community. These local conditions may have helped to create a perceived safer environment to be open about HIV. Another possibility was that because more of the interviewees in Miami discussed living in poverty they may have felt they had less to lose by disclosing. Interestingly, those who were open about their status shared entrepreneurial characteristics. They had been living with HIV for decades, accepted HIV, and had a high drive to be active and to create productive enterprises, which may have empowered them to be open about HIV and to withstand the social judgment and discrimination their HIV status exposed them to.

A constellation of life experiences, personal characteristics, and social networks came together to support the decision to be open about HIV. Length of time since diagnosis could play a role in this decision because acceptance did have a temporal dimension. However, time was not sufficient in creating openness about HIV because some participants who were living with HIV for years were not open about their HIV. Being creative, active, social, wanting to shine in the world, and to create a legacy were related to being open, but were not sufficient because other participants such as Walter and Chris had these characteristics and yet they were not open about their HIV, potentially because they had not yet fully adjusted to their new lives with HIV and had been diagnosed for only one year. Walter was in denial of his HIV and emphasized his belief that his contacts in the music industry would not accept his HIV and that if he were open about HIV he would lose his reputation and career. Chris worked as a teacher and also feared being open because he worked with children. Perhaps the quality of social contacts and the social context of the type of industry and profession were related to the decision to disclose.

Another difference may be that unlike Chris and Walter, those who ran their own businesses may have thus had more freedom to make the life altering decision to be open about their HIV because they felt less dependent on others for employment. An entrepreneur mindset involves the ability to take calculated risks, to work in a context of uncertainty and to navigate new social terrains, a strong belief in the self and one's abilities, a high level of discipline and intrinsic motivation, drive to succeed, and passion for work. Being open about HIV was a calculated risk that was taken and negotiated by launching new businesses and being flexible in approaches to work by adapting to create new businesses. They created these new projects by using their entrepreneurial skills as they worked to withstand the rejection and judgment of others by harnessing their strong beliefs in their work and themselves. Autonomy in work could have influenced the decision to be open about HIV, allowing for more flexibility in work opportunities, as opposed to someone dependent on an occupational institution for employment and mobility. For example, Chris had less freedom working as teacher. Chris still worked to leave a legacy by helping the children he worked with but worked to leave this legacy in secret and was dependent on his employer to do his work. Sarah was the only self-reported entrepreneur in the Frankfurt sample. However, she was not open about her HIV and reported that she could not disclose due to her living conditions because she lived in a small German town where she would be exposed to gossip and chose to hide her HIV. In contrast, living in a more liberal and urban area may provide a greater feeling of anonymity and freedom, which may have helped to create a social context where being open about HIV was perceived as more of an opportunity then as a barrier to creative production and work.

As Schütz (1962) theorized, social interaction involves an element of threat or danger because it is in a constant state of flux. Furthermore, it can be argued that danger allows for change and change allows for agency and action. The delicate nature of interaction as being fluid allows for action because it provides the opportunity to change one's life. The threat in interaction can be a powerful opportunity. If we are aware of our potential in each moment, and are attuned to the fluidity and malleability in interaction, this allows into awareness our ability to shape reality. Realization of the power to fundamentally alter social relations starting with influencing social interactions can provide the opportunity to act upon this realization to counter existing negative stereotypes of HIV. This highlights the importance of being open about HIV and acting to challenge negative stereotypes. Therefore, the discussion of being open about HIV and acting to raise awareness about HIV, and to help others with HIV among the Miami sample is important in understanding how PLWHA can act to improve not only their own personal lives, but the lives of others with HIV, and how they can act to alter local conceptions of illness. As demonstrated in the Frankfurt sample, disclosure can be seen as a decision that involves a consideration of social losses and rejection. In the Frankfurt sample, HIV was often discussed as a "secret" that could not be told.

Perhaps due to the different types of interviews used for each sample, the processes involved in the decision to disclose were made more visible in the narrative interviews than in the topical interviews. This difference may also be due to the lack of openness about HIV status among the Frankfurt sample, which made issues related to the decision to disclose more prominent than in the Miami sample. The Miami sample was characterized by more openness about HIV status and also by more reports of working to create social change for people living with HIV and to increase other's awareness. Being open about HIV can allow for the expansion of social worlds, increasing resources and discourse, thus increasing power. Openness about HIV can create the opportunity for gaining power, reclaiming social status and legitimacy, and influencing the working world by engaging in collective social action to change common discourse about HIV. HIV was described as faceless, or not being represented in public discourse. Openness and raising awareness of HIV and of coming out about HIV allowed for the creation of a face of HIV that countered the negative social stereotypes about people with HIV. HIV was described as being faceless and lacking representation and coming out about HIV allowed for representation.

By giving a face to HIV, HIV was taken out of the shadows of the figurative closet and given form in the working world expanding the social world of HIV. HIV was not seen as represented in public discourse, which rendered the images surrounding HIV as shadowy, amorphous, ambiguous, marginalized, deviant, and contested. This excerpt also emphasized the difficulties that people with HIV living in small towns can face. Isolation and secrecy in being unable to disclose was related the social context of neighborhoods and the spatial limitations of not having HIV services and support groups close by. Rural versus urban communities and their spatial and neighborhood conditions appeared to contextualize life experiences of living with HIV in both samples.

3.9.2   "Ethical Persuasion":
A Technique for the Management of Social Interaction

Walter protected his secret with what he called "ethical persuasion" in conversation Walter's discussion of "ethical persuasion" provided insight into techniques that can be used in daily social interaction in order to maintain the secret of HIV. Walter described how his diagnosis "threw" him into a split, heroic identity. He presented an image of himself as Superman and living a double life, this double life involved the image of heroism and of strength. This maintained Walter's view of himself as autonomous, masculine, and strong. Walter's diagnosis threw him into a double life, into a split in identity. On one side of a door that could not be opened, resided a hero who carried with strength the burden of an unknown dark secret. On the other side, was a man who was "normal." Walter explained that he negotiated this split identity and double life by using "ethical persuasion":

> "How do I deal with it? (laughs) I mean (-) that's (--) that's a good question (laughs) that's a good question I how do I deal with it? I mean (-) well you know (-) I just um (--) see um ethical persuasion you know (-) and I ethically persuade in certain (---) situations where I (-) you know ok if a conversations sort of leaning this way let me intervene and kinda push it this way so that we don't go this way know what I mean? Um again (-) I'm not (--) I'm a pretty informed person about a lot of things (-) uh yeah I'm aware of a few things (-) let's put it like that and um even when it deals with um ending (uv) and talking and um verbal and things (--) I'm (-) I can deal with these certain (-) I know how to (-) I understand these certain things so I just kinda (-) you know (-) control it and take it somewhere else. I can't tell you how. I just have to be in that situation (-) to explain that, you know, so I can't really tell you how I do it (-) it's just that (-) it just happens." [Transcript 1, lines 487-499]

"Ethical persuasion" involved moving the conversation subtly away from any hints of his identity as being HIV-positive and was a means of controlling social interaction. However, this act of "ethical persuasion" had implications for Walter's identity as he perceived himself as "real" as an honest person. Therefore, this action could create a conflict in his life, potentially shifting his self-conception of himself as a hero into a villain who repulses himself because of his actions that counter his conceptions of virtue by contradicting his value of being "real." Walter associated impression management work in hiding HIV as a means of "coping" with HIV, suggesting that while he denied the existence of HIV on an emotional level, he felt that he coped in an active way by engaging in ethical persuasion, which paradoxically served to deny and hide the existence of HIV to others.

Walter could not articulate exactly how he performed ethical persuasion. Rather, it was an act which "just happens" which suggests that ethical persuasion was fluent and subconscious in his social interactions. Interestingly, ethical persuasion was an active method of coping and yet involved action taken at avoidance of the issue of HIV. Both Rachel and Walter discussed means of avoidance, Rachel engaged in physical avoidance of others when she felt stigmatized and Walter uses linguistic avoidance of the topic of HIV.

Therefore, the use of "ethical persuasion" involved Walter's use of agency, of actively shaping social interaction and acting to shape his circumstances. However, this expression of agency denied a part of his identity because he was a "real" person" and hated fake people. So Walter was sacrificing parts of his self to maintain secrecy. At the time of the interview, he preferred be fake than to be defined as a disease so that he could maintain his image of strength, intelligence, and sexual attractiveness. Living a double life involved a split awareness, and rendered HIV unreal, but also served to protect the self from societal judgment and potential rejection. Why was it a door which could not be opened? Walter felt that in order to maintain his secret he had to violate principles that he valued. The case of Walter demonstrates how zero or nondisclosure can be paralyzing and can forgo possibilities of support and personal development and receiving help, and resources. Negotiating social worlds appeared to be easier when participants had a supportive reaction to their disclosure. However, in order to be open to the possibility of a supportive reaction, participants had to be willing to risk disclosure.

Being cautious and feeling threatened due to the maintenance of secrecy was stressful and could be a process that can create conditions for stress proliferation (Pearlin et al. 2005). Maintaining the secret of HIV with nondisclosure can create additional social strain. While the concept of coping is often associated with psychology, negotiating the strain or stress of HIV is a sociological concern as it involves processes related to adjustment to new social roles, identity, labeling, deviance, and stress resulting from strain. Indeed, stress research in sociology can be traced back to Merton's (1938) work on social structure and anomie or "strain theory" and to Merton's (1957) emphasis on role strain. More contemporary work on the sociological study of stress such as the work of Pearlin (1989), Aneshensel (1992), and others (Turner et al. 1995) has further developed the processes and concepts involved in the stress process with an emphasis on the intersectionality of social positions, resources, a refinement of multiple types of stress and stressors, elaboration of mediators and moderators in the stress process, roles, role sets, and how role expectations alter interpersonal relations and can therefore lead to stress.

Prior research demonstrates that HIV disclosure, when the reaction to disclosure is supportive, is significantly associated with higher immune functioning and a lower viral load and that this relationship involves a reduction in stress (Fekete et al. 2009). Qualitative research has also found that disclosure was related to social support and positive adjustment to HIV (Medley et al. 2009). Therefore, under supportive conditions, disclosure may serve as a means of reducing the strain of maintaining the secrecy of HIV. Because disclosure, stress, and stigma are interrelated and rooted in historical and personal biographies, my analysis builds on the suggestions of prior researchers in sociology to more fully examine the stress process as rooted in life experience and social context.

3.9.3   Fear of Rejection

Because of the awareness of stigma, disclosure may be seen as a decision where actors consider the social losses and consequences of disclosure. This awareness manifested itself in participants' discussions of their fears of rejection, negotiation of social interaction to avoid being identified as being HIV-positive, and the separation of social worlds (HIV-positive versus HIV-negative). Fear of sexual rejection appeared to be related to disclosure to sexual partners. Interestingly, Chris chose to avoid unsafe sexual contact but still maintained his secret of HIV, as compared to Walter who engaged in sexual contact without disclosing and who also engaged in unprotected sex. Both men felt that disclosure to a sexual partner was difficult but Chris refrained from sex with someone who was HIV-negative. What accounted for this difference? Perhaps because Chris was in a committed, loving relationship he did not feel the need to engage in sex with other partners and so it was easier for him to keep distance from other sexual partners. Another factor that may explain this difference is that Chris accepted that risky sexual behavior led to his HIV status whereas Walter was in denial.

In contrast to Walter, Nancy disclosed to her husband at the time of her diagnosis. Nancy insisted on using protection because she wanted to have a child and felt that if she or her husband were to get sick they would not be able to take care of a child. Sarah did not discuss any sexual contact with her deceased husband or any other sexual behavior. Rachel described that her reason for HIV disclosure to her boyfriend was her pregnancy and she did not disclose until after engaging in unprotected sex with her partner. George also disclosed to his partner at the time of his HIV diagnosis and felt that his husband was at first shocked but learned to deal with HIV. George explained that because he and his partner had been to being together for twenty years, sexual contact was not as frequent. George felt that because of their infrequent sexual encounters HIV was not as major of an issue in their relationship. George cheated on his partner with another man and had to disclose his HIV status to this man and felt that it was embarrassing but necessary and practiced safe sex.

David engaged in safe sex but trusted one of his sexual partners enough to not use a condom. David did not discuss his current sexual behavior so it was unclear if he was sexually active. However, David described his lifestyle as being characterized by moderation and careful behavior. David believed that as long as people took their medication and as long as they lived healthy lifestyles, they could have a normal life. David emphasized that people with HIV could have a glass of wine or a beer, "normal day life," but not above the limit, they could have a regular life (Sequential Report 8, p. 6). This suggested that David lived a life of moderation and was mindful of his health and the health of others. Moderation and caution were important aspects of negotiating social relationships and daily life.

Fear of rejection upon HIV disclosure was discussed by Chris who Chris delved deeper into the issue of being gay and the questions related to HIV that parents ask their children come out about their sexuality. Chris related this to his own experience of disclosing his HIV status to his mother. Here Chris rendered dialogue and described how he reassured his mother that he would not die and how now at the end of the interview his mother had accepted his HIV. Chris then returned to the topic of not being able to tell his friend who was romantically interested in him that he had HIV because he was not sure how they would react. Chris emphasized that he would rather have a supportive friendship than to lose the relationship due to disclosing his status. Chris did not want to "take the chance" or "risk" losing his friend so he chose to keep his HIV status private. He elaborated:

> "One thing I would be scared of is to be rejected and um to not be supported just because I'm having HIV like everyone's really supportive now uhm but like I said when people don't know how to…deal with certain things they run off because they're scared um (--) and yeah (--) that's probably one of my worst fears (--) to be rejected and not have anyone to turn to but like the disease itself is not really a problem for me (long pause) any further questions?" [Transcript 3, lines 121-133]

Chris revealed that rejection was one of his "worst fears." Chris said that everyone was currently supportive but the fear of being isolated and losing that support was a major fear. After approaching his deep fear of rejection, Chris closed the interview. Why did Chris emphasize that HIV was a nonissue for him after he revealed that his worst fear was rejection due to HIV disclosure? Perhaps, Chris while on the surface appeared to be doing well, still wrestled with unresolved dilemmas in regards to his fear of rejection. Although Chris felt loved, had access to medication, and was healthy, his fear of stigma appeared to still be an unresolved dilemma. Why did Chris end his narrative in this way? Perhaps he coped by staying active, social, and positive and wanted to be seen in a positive light so when his deepest fears surfaced he made sure to say that HIV was not an issue and moved away from a discussion of this fear. Fear of rejection was prevalent in the cases analyzed, suggesting that this fear of rejection was important in shaping participants' experiences despite their diverse backgrounds.

Fear of rejection seemed to coincide with decisions related to disclosure because both Walter and Chris discussed rejection as it could occur in the context of sexual partnerships. Walter emphasized that disclosing his HIV during sex would lead to rejection. This was a critical moment in Walter's interview as he asked me what I would do if someone disclosed their HIV status to me during a sexual encounter. Walter's question was literal and Walter probed for an answer before continuing his interview. The issue of HIV disclosure affecting sexual encounters and relationships was important to Walter. He emphasized the moment right before the decision to have sex with a partner. The moment was stressed. What would happen in that moment if he were to disclose? He felt that if he were to disclose his HIV status this moment would be shattered and sex would not occur. Kissing was discussed as "emotional contact" and as not being purely physical or sexual. For Walter, kissing was not the relevant issue, sexual intercourse was. He continued:

> "It won't happen for one (-) that person will not have sex and two now you're a contagious disease. (-) not only that, that person will tell her circle who will tell that circle and then it spreads before you know you gotta run outta town (-) move to another state (-) or another country or something or a little bit further away because (-) you know what I'm saying, now you're looked at as some type of outcast (-) so to speak you know what I mean? Again I can't do that, you know what I'm saying? My intention wasn't to just have sex with these women and you know infect them also kept that in (-) I'm not trying to infect nobody if it's true that I have this I'm not out to infect anybody as um like (-) I'm not like that (-) I'm not a murderer." [Transcript 1, lines 688-708]

Walter maintained that the "average person" would bring up a series of questions. First, the HIV disclosure would take away the possibility of sexual intercourse. Secondly, disclosure was seen as having more widespread consequences. HIV disclosure would serve to redefine Walter from a potential sexual partner to a "contagious disease." Walter feared telling the women he slept with about his HIV status because he did not trust that his secret would be kept in confidence. Rather, Walter expected for the information regarding his HIV status to spread across networks of people until he would be forced to leave his social surroundings because once everyone knew he had HIV he would be defined as an "outcast." Therefore, Walter was aware of the stigma attached to HIV and worked to avoid experiencing social distance and rejection. He did not want his reputation as a musician or as an attractive sexual partner to be affected so he decided to keep his HIV status a secret. For Walter, his own self-preservation and legitimacy were more salient in the decision to disclose than any feelings of responsibility for infecting others. His construction of HIV as an experiment may also have served to support his reasons for not disclosing because if HIV was not truly real, then there was no need to disclose.

This suggested that when addressing the issue of safe sexual behavior and HIV disclosure to sexual partners, it was important to understand the fear that people with HIV can face in having to reveal a status that they feel will lead to social rejection and exclusion. Also, denial of HIV status may prevent HIV disclosure to sexual partners. Walter claimed that he was not deliberately trying to give anyone HIV. He emphasized multiple times that his intention was not to infect others with HIV. However, Walter realized that while what he was doing was dangerous he was not a "murderer." Walter was aware of the potential harm of unprotected sex but because he felt that he lacked the intention to infect others, he felt he was not to blame for their possible infection. There also remained an element of doubt of the existence of HIV as he added "if it's true that I have this." HIV appeared to be on the edge of Walter's awareness because he recognized the harm that could result from risky sexual behavior but pushed this possibility out of his awareness by arguing that he just trying to protect himself from rejection. Walter was aware of HIV transmission but did not use condoms and did not disclose, which indicated that an awareness of the modes of HIV transmission was not sufficient in preventing the transmission of HIV. Sexual practices need to be contextualized in terms of the meaning and importance sex and intimacy have in order to be relevant.

Unlike Walter, Rachel chose to tell the person she was sexually intimate that she had HIV. For example, Rachel elaborated on how telling her boyfriend was difficult. Initially, she did not tell her boyfriend about her HIV. When Rachel became pregnant, this made her feel that she needed to disclose her status. Due to being pregnant and having HIV, there were certain medical precautions that had to be taken in order to prevent HIV transmission to her child. Therefore, Rachel felt that her boyfriend had to know the truth. However, before this she explicitly stated that she did not tell him because she was afraid. If Rachel had not become pregnant, she may have never disclosed her HIV status to her partner.

Fears of rejection were not unfounded. David experienced an involuntary disclosure of his HIV status when a local newspaper covered the story of his HIV activism. David specifically asked for his identity to be protected but the story was identifiable and his status was made public against his will. David experienced many people withdrawing and rejecting him after his HIV was made public in the newspaper. Therefore, fear of rejection was grounded in real life consequences of social exclusion. Interestingly, Rachel did not explicitly discuss fear of rejection in a sexual context. Rachel did not disclose her HIV status to her boyfriend until after she was pregnant suggesting that she also had unprotected sex without disclosing. Rachel emphasized the fear of being seen using HIV services or taking her medication by others and did not discuss her sexual behavior. Maintaining the secret of HIV was also an especially important issue for gay respondents because of the close associations between conceptions of HIV and homosexuality.

3.9.4   Support and HIV Disclosure

HIV disclosure emerged as an important facet of participants' experiences and was interrelated with action, social support, and stigma. Disclosure can enhance coping by increasing social support and helping people to take action in order to overcome a trajectory of suffering. The reactions of others to disclosure can either confirm or disconfirm negative expectations, either enhancing feelings of support and agency, or alternatively increasing levels of stigma and shame. Disclosure and action appeared to share a reciprocal relationship, which could be conceptualized as a feedback loop. For example, action manifested itself at times in the decision to disclosure and disclosure in turn reduced stigma. Reductions in stigma then feedback into enhancing action by reducing fear of detection, increasing control over life circumstances such as treatment, relationships with others, and reducing the burden of secrecy. Participants disclosed to intimate partners, family members, or to other patients. For example, when Rachel was diagnosed her only family in her native country was her elderly grandmother who lived far away. Rachel's mother contacted her from Germany and Rachel described how she told her mother everything because she felt certain that only her mother could understand her problems. Similarly, Chris felt he received love and support upon his disclosure to his partner. Strong, loving relationships helped Chris to cope with his new life with HIV. Chris had taken strides in resolving his struggles with HIV due to his partner's acceptance. Faced with a new identity as being HIV-positive, Chris' conception of himself as he knew it broke down and he was confronted with a new possibility that he could be a danger to his partner's health. However, because his partner accepted him despite his diagnosis, Chris was able to resolve this existential struggle and to maintain his relationship. Therefore, receiving love and acceptance can be instrumental in overcoming deeply rooted existential and social relationship crises.

Participants reported selective disclosure. Often they disclosed only to family, friends, intimate partners, or to some combination of these groups. Those that reported disclosure to friends emphasized the closeness of their friendships and chose to disclose selectively to about zero to three friends. Experiencing a positive, accepting, and supportive reaction upon HIV disclosure was reported as helpful to participants. In the context of the heavy burden of maintaining a "double life" or the "secret" of HIV, this suggested that acceptance upon disclosure can lessen the burden of maintaining a life of secrecy in the face of illness. The decision to disclose was carefully considered by participants. Another condition affecting the decision to disclose was if they had experienced a severely deteriorated health status where their lives were in danger and they were in need of help.

Therefore, while not generalizable, the relationship of disclosure and coping can be conceptualized as a process. First, considerations of the reactions by others to disclosure were negotiated in assessing the social risk involved in disclosure. Next, if the relationship with the person to disclose to was considered safe enough, or if it was deemed necessary to disclose, the decision to engage in disclosure was made. After disclosure, the reactions of others played an essential role because these reactions either confirmed a negative expectation or a positive one. A positive reaction to HIV disclosure, such as in the case of Sarah where both her children and therapist reacted supportively, can provide a sense of support and understanding, lessening the burden of the secret of HIV and facilitating an awareness of inner strength and action. Conversely, a negative reaction could further isolate and confirm negative expectations of people's attitudes towards HIV. Participants in both samples emphasized the importance of normalcy in their relationships after disclosure. Therefore, a positive reaction that did not undermine the nature of social relationships was reported as highly valued by participants. Also, PLWHA may experience a range of negative to positive reactions from others and the more people they disclose to, the higher the chance of both reactions. For example, David disclosed to three close friends and experienced a positive reaction. However, he reported that:

"It is always heavy this secret, this is heavy because you always think 'They might find out' you're very careful to speak about things. Well the interesting thing is I started speaking about HIV very often with families and friends, since I started this program, but the rationale is they listened, but they never came back or they never asked back or whatever. I don't know why, I never found out why. Probably, probably they don't want to get in touch with that. This is a very interesting eh, eh subject I guess, one of the biggest pieces. They just listen 'Oh ok, ok' that's it."
[Sequential Report 8, p. 3 f.]

David actively discussed HIV to communities in order to increase HIV awareness but the reactions of others to this information indicated to him that people
listened but did not appear to be open, concerned, or accepting about the issue of
HIV. The evasive attitudes of others towards HIV were problematic for David
and "one of the biggest pieces" of the puzzle of understanding public views of
HIV. Participants made a distinction between the public and personal spheres of
their lives. HIV was often described as not being other people's "business" and
participants were very cautious in maintaining their secret of HIV from coworkers,
employers, and acquaintances. However, in the private sphere of friends and
family, disclosure often had a positive effect leading to support and
understanding.

3.9.5   *The Decision to Disclose: A Consideration of Social Losses and Rejection*

The decision to disclose was a difficult decision that involved a consideration of
social consequences. Specifically, potential social losses and rejection were major
considerations as participants made decisions to disclosure. The anticipation of
rejection and severed social ties highlighted the role of anticipated stigma in HIV
disclosure. As Lemert (1974) argued, other's reactions to a deviant status, or
societal reaction, are a major factor in the social construction of deviance. At the
interactional level, disclosure can facilitate a major change in social interaction
by either confirming or disproving expectations of other's behavior. Disclosure,
stigma, and social support must be examined in relation to one another. For
example, Rachel described her reasons for telling her boyfriend about her HIV
status, which allowed her to receive support from her boyfriend but also exposed
her to stigma by her boyfriend's mother. Rachel told her boyfriend because she
felt that she wanted to have a monogamous and serious relationship with her
boyfriend and not "go on looking for one man to the next."

The reactions of others were also important to Chris. Chris contextualized his
decisions regarding HIV disclosure as having social costs in the form of potential
lost social ties with others. Chris was sensitive to an "inherent danger in
interaction" due to his HIV because he was aware of how his HIV disclosure could
redefine his social relations and interactions (Strauss 1997). Chris revealed that
rejection was one of his "worst fears." Chris felt supported but being isolated and
losing that support was a major fear. Fear of rejection was more important to
Chris than the physical aspects of HIV. The power of stigma, the stress stigma
put on decisions to disclose, and the costs of having to maintain a secret of HIV

were emergent themes in all cases analyzed. Sarah waited over a decade to disclose to her sons and has only disclosed to three close friends, including her sister who was a physician. Sarah disclosed her status immediately upon her discovery of HIV to only one confidant, she waited years to disclose to the others. The decision to disclose was a conscious deliberation that involved considerations of potential social losses and loss of social status as Sarah explained:

"I didn't tell anybody (-) that was the next thing (-) because talking about stigma that was in those times especially. And I was younger myself also you're not as self-competent (-) intelligent as you are twenty years later (-) and so I just made up my mind "I won't tell anybody" this is my thing so I did (-) so still nobody knows." [Transcript 5, lines 37-46]

Despite the enormity of her confrontation with HIV, Sarah chose to keep her HIV diagnosis to herself and to not disclose. Sarah used the term "stigma" emphasizing how anticipation of stigma influenced her decision to not disclose. Sarah also made a distinction between the social context of HIV back in the early 1990s and in the present at the time of the interview. Sarah felt that in the past there was a great amount of stigma surrounding HIV. Importantly, her discussion of stigma was rooted in historical perspective and in the context of fear of HIV in the 1990s, illustrating how stigma cannot be divorced from its historical context. She also explained a temporal difference in her self-view. Sarah used her conception of time to relate to herself and to situate her story which was illustrative of Husserl's (1964) notion of the key role of temporality in being and the reflexive nature of the "dasein" as being oriented towards the nature of its being in time. Sarah felt that in the past she was younger, less "self-competent" and "intelligent" than she felt twenty years later. Sarah also described her decision to not disclose as another conscious choice of her own deliberation.

Sarah waited over a decade to tell her children that she had HIV. She described her children's shock, which she expected and this was part of the reason that she waited to tell them. Sarah waited until her children were older, until they were farther along in their education. This indicated a great consideration of her children's emotions and well-being because she took a great effort to maintain this secret until her children had reached an age where she felt that they would be able to handle her disclosure. Also, Sarah's husband died and so she was a single parent trying to raise her children, manage her HIV, and maintain her secret of HIV. Her children lost their father at a young age and Sara may have felt protective of their feelings and attuned to their needs, which also contributed to her not disclosing until they were much older. This indicated a great deal of responsibility that required an enormous amount of inner resolve and strength and yet she did not dwell on the work she did to maintain her life and the lives of her children for all these years.

In contrast to Sarah, George immediately disclosed to his husband and to his family. George described his husband reacting with shock and said that it was the only time he saw his husband cry. George's husband was not in Germany, George called him and his husband's reaction was described as being very serious. At first, George's husband was scared of contracting HIV and would be fearful if George was bleeding but George felt that this was no longer a problem a year later. However, George's husband did not like to speak about HIV and they did not have sex often.

George discussed his disclosure to his family, particularly to his mother, who he described as "super mama" (Sequential Report 7, p. 4). George was unsure if he would live to be eighty or ninety years old, he did not expect to live this long because the medication is still new and no one knows the long-term effects. George's mother was fearful that he would die but George felt that everyone dies and this was something his mother needed to accept. George needed to comfort his mother; it was hard for his mother to accept that HIV was his problem, not her problem. George felt supported by his mother, they supported each other, and he described their relationship as a "give and take" (Sequential Report 7, p. 4). George did not know what it would be like without his family and felt that the support of his family was important. Despite their acceptance, George reported feelings of embarrassment at having to reveal the secret of having HIV because they asked him how he contracted HIV and his mother and husband discovered that he had another man in his life sexually because the issue of HIV raised questions about his sexual behavior.

Disclosure, when it lead to the attainment of understanding and support, and did not change the nature of social relationships in a fundamentally negative way, enhanced feelings of support. However, the decision to disclose is itself an important emergent phenomenon, which involved a substantial amount of work and a consideration of social losses. A fear of rejection, anticipated stigma, a desire to maintain social status and to protect one's reputation, and the consideration of other's emotions such as in the case of Sarah who waited until her children were eighteen and in the case of Arthur who did not tell his mother, were all major considerations which influenced the decision to disclose.

Therefore, other's reactions to HIV disclosure as positive and supportive versus negative and isolating served to confirm and disconfirm fears of rejection, setting the stage for future social interaction. Disclosure had the potential to fundamentally change social relationships. The current analysis, rooted in the personal and collective histories of participants, grounds an analysis of deviance in an "ethnographic present" and in history, helping to address the criticism of labeling theory as being "astructural and ahistorical" (Lemert 1981). By focusing on the decision to disclose and by examining the interrelations between action, disclosure, and stigma a deeper insight was gained into how societal reaction and the anticipation of this reaction shapes action for those with a deviant status. The anticipation of other's reaction, or of societal reaction as termed by Lemert (1974), and as emphasized in more contemporary labeling theory, emerged as an important factor related to disclosure and to the anticipation of stigma.

3.9.6   *Stigma: Appearance, Privacy, and Visibility*

3.9.6.1   Anticipated Stigma

The anticipation of stigma appeared to be rooted in conceptions of how society categorized people with HIV. The anticipation of stigma corresponded to the concept of felt stigma (Jacoby 1994; Scambler 2004). In accordance with modified labeling theory, social meanings ascribed to HIV were internalized by participants as they discussed their understanding of public conceptions of HIV (Link et al. 1989). The struggle of integrating negative conceptions associated with HIV into their self-concepts emphasized the problematic aspects involved in the internalization of negative stereotypes of HIV. Processes related to the internalization of stigma were rooted in moral discourse. Participants associated HIV with images of drug addiction, sexual deviance, irresponsibility, and marginalized social status. In addition, when making sense of existing and new conceptions of HIV, participants both recently diagnosed with HIV and those living with HIV for long periods of time made comparisons between HIV, cancer, and other chronic illnesses. The stress and isolation of living in secret with HIV was expressed profoundly when Sarah described her uterus cancer as a relaxation in comparison to HIV:

> "I was operated and uh uterus cancer (-) ah well that was (-) on the other hand (-) somehow a sort of relaxation you know (-) because cancer you can tell anyone (-) and [...] everyone wants to help you (-) wants to be of support (-) or whatever and that was why I say it was a sort of a relaxation because there was something you could talk about." [Transcript 5, lines 86-91]

This emphasizes how disclosure can provide relief and support in the face of illness. Furthermore, this demonstrates how the anticipation of stigma can be a major barrier for patients, preventing them from obtaining support in the face of illness. Sarah felt that with her cancer she could be open and that people were supportive. Her conceptualization of cancer as a relaxation emphasized the untold burden involved in Sarah's maintenance of her secret of HIV. With cancer, she could disclose her illness without social judgment and in return she received support, which was helpful to her in this critical moment for her health. The anticipated stigma of her HIV prevented her from disclosing. Thus, her anticipation of stigma prevented her from obtaining support both during her initial diagnosis and throughout her life as she continuously worked to keep HIV a secret. Sarah discussed another recent health problem, a stroke.

Only a few months before our interview, Sarah had a stroke. She minimized the magnitude of the stroke by adding that it was "very light" but she was hospitalized for a week. Sarah compared this to the time she was in the hospital for cancer, similar to her experience with her operation, the stroke prompted her friends to come to the hospital and to show their support in her time of need. She contrasted this with HIV as she explained that "HIV is still secret." Sarah did not expect to receive a similar reaction to her HIV as she did with her cancer and stroke, which further illustrated her anticipation of HIV stigma. Similarly, Chris emphasized a difference between public views of HIV and cancer:

"Everyone knows about cancer and everyone knows yeah there's this big um right of cancer (-) types you know so it's not that big of a deal but if someone hears 'HIV' or AIDS it's just like 'oh wow no omg it's like death (-) end of the world' that reaction should be like (--) shouldn't be like that not these days anymore (-) cause there's so many people doing so much work and putting so much effort into it for negative people to understand and see that it's just a disease like everything else you know it's not like you're gonna die if you shake my hand or stuff like that just to (--) not even be (-) I don't want people to um be understanding or to accept or whatever just to **know** that it's (-) you're not gonna die by talking to me or drinking out of my cup or something like that." [Transcript 3, lines 258-269]

Chris was aware of anti-stigma movements for HIV and efforts to promote understanding of HIV but he felt that these efforts were not effective in reducing stigma and reducing the public's fears and misconceptions of HIV. An awareness of the fear of HIV transmission was acknowledged as a cause of distinction in the conceptions of cancer and HIV. Chris explained that people were aware and informed about cancer but that HIV was associated with a fear of contagion and death. For Chris, HIV represented a hidden stigma, which involved a double awareness of being treated normal and yet knowing that he could be treated much differently. Chris overheard discussions of HIV and felt that people were shallow but justified their "ignorance" by explaining his views of HIV prior to his diagnosis. This allowed for a justification of others' misconceptions of HIV, serving to minimize the discomfort of observing misconceptions about HIV. Overhearing negative discussions of HIV by others was described by other participants. For example, Walter described what it was like for him to overhear his coworkers talk about HIV:

> "There's a lot of (pause) uniformed people, they don't know about this disease you know 'Oh you have HIV oh you're gonna die in a couple years, stay away from me, you're contagious' (-) know what I'm saying? Its (--) there's people out there like this you know what I mean? I'm around people, [...] I'm around people they even (-) you know they talk about this, I hear about this but I say nothing (-) I just listen 'Really? Wow, interesting' (-) I hear what they say. I can't say nothing to these people. You know this (-) this (-) this (-) this is a dark secret that I have to take to the grave with me." [Transcript 1, lines 460-473]

Similar to Chris, Walter felt that other's fear of HIV infection, views of HIV as a deadly, infectious disease, and lack of knowledge were factors contributing to negative attitudes towards HIV. Walter felt that HIV disclosure would put him at risk of social rejection and of being redefined as a contagious disease. David also compared his perception of public views of cancer and HIV. David discussed how HIV was more feared by the public than cancer even though cancer can be more deadly than HIV. According to David, cancer could be discussed openly and accepted but HIV was a taboo subject and had to be kept secret. David tried to understand where this fear of HIV came from and did not feel that education was enough to reduce negative views of HIV because he had seen people that were very well-educated have negative attitudes towards HIV. David emphasized that despite having education and understanding how HIV is transmitted, those with high educational attainment could still hold negative attitudes. David experienced fearful reactions by physicians and other professionals both in treatment and in his personal life. Accordingly, he felt that education and information were not enough to reduce public misconceptions and fear of HIV. David also grounded HIV stigma in historical context. For David, age and generational factors were perceived as playing a role in shaping views of HIV. David believed that younger people who were not exposed to the HIV panic in the 1980s and 1990s were more tolerant and less fearful of HIV.

Nancy also anticipated a stigmatizing reaction to HIV disclosure due to negative public stereotypes of HIV. Nancy explained that people talked about HIV like a deadly disease, that she was scared that people would see her going to the doctor, and she did not feel comfortable seeking care. Nancy was fearful that maybe someone from work or from her country would see her and then someone would talk about her sickness to others. Nancy felt that this was a fear that many people have. Indeed, other participants reported either a fear of gossip or experienced gossip about their health. Prior research has identified gossip as a type of "verbal stigma" of HIV (Cao et al. 2006). Verbal stigma or gossip was a central concern for participants who felt that gossip was a dangerous form of social exclusion that had the power to discredit them and to spread negative attitudes towards them to a larger social network. Gossip was a major concern and fear among participants that placed their social relationships, careers, and legitimacy at risk and had the power to socially isolate and ostracize them.

Nancy anticipated stigma because she had heard stories from others who had been rejected due to HIV. Nancy had a great deal of fear of being identified as being HIV-positive prior to her engagement in Helping Hand. Initially, her anticipation of stigma prevented her from seeking support from Helping Hand. The doctors at the clinic told Nancy to meet the other patients at Helping Hand but Nancy was afraid to go because she was not sure who she would see at the meetings. Nancy explained:

> "You are always living in fear (-) like when you are coming here it is like living in fear let me not see someone who knows me." (Sequential Report 6, p. 3).

Being seen seeking services was a risk many participants were cautious to take due to a fear of exposure of their HIV status. Participants expressed a deep fear of gossip unmasking their secret of HIV and thus rendering them as social outcasts. This suggests a dialectic where access to a supportive, safe community of similar others can contribute to feelings of empowerment and reduce fear. Yet fear of detection and anticipation of stigma were major barriers preventing participation in Helping Hand in the first place.

In order to overcome and eliminate stigma, participation in groups such as Helping Hand can provide valuable resources. Psychosocial resources such as social support can increase feelings of self-efficacy and information about treatment, and this in turn can provide access to additional resources. For example, some participants became active in the HIV community and their activism was related to their membership in Helping Hand, which enhanced their feelings of being able to spread awareness about HIV. Therefore, processes of group identification, acceptance, and action can operate to reduce stigma. However, a dialectic emerged where in order to overcome stigma, participants had to overcome their fear of rejection and anticipation of stigma, risking their relationships and status. In order to combat stigma this fear of stigma must be resolved. Resolution of this conflict could potentially involve either initiatives targeting people with HIV and involving them in anti-stigma efforts while making participants comfortable and protecting their HIV status. Or, more radically, people being open with their HIV status and turning what was a source of oppression into power could help to facilitate social change. Because of the devastating social losses related to disclosure, legal protection could enable people with HIV to feel more comfortable in revealing their status and to protect them from discrimination. The consequences of stigma were very powerful determinants preventing participants from being open about their HIV status. For example, Arthur anticipated stigma and so he chose to not disclose his HIV status:

> "When I was diagnosed with HIV (-) I lived like a closeted life (-) nobody knew just younger members of the family knew about me being gay and also being infected I didn't tell anyone at work (-) uh (--) well I kept it like in the closet because I didn't want them to know because I think I would have had problems at work (-) I used to work at [...] at a kind of good position there as well (-) uh I thought it was not (-) not (-) not good for my future career to come out with the infection as well." [Transcript 4, lines 22-29]

Arthur described his initial life with HIV as being a "closeted life" and only the younger members of his family knew about his sexual orientation and his HIV status. Perhaps because he was an older white European man, he came from a family with a more conservative background and felt that the younger members of his family were more accepting of his sexuality and HIV than more traditional family members. This suggests that there may be a generational aspect to disclosure and stigma because disclosure can be dependent on the age group with which one identifies and older generations may not understand the dilemmas of their newer generation.

Importantly, Arthur discussed his work conditions. Arthur felt that HIV disclosure would be detrimental to his future career and anticipated difficulties if he were to disclose. Therefore, Arthur was aware of HIV stigma and because of this anticipated stigma he chose to keep his HIV private. Work was an important theme in his narrative. The importance of work and nondisclosure in occupational settings was also emphasized in the other cases. For example, Chris emphasized the importance of helping others through his role as a teacher. Sarah discussed the value of being well-respected in her profession, and Walter emphasized his need to be respected as a musician. Participants reported a deep fear of losing their legitimacy in their chosen professions and a fear of losing their jobs upon HIV disclosure. Therefore, participants had to negotiate the critical issue of feeling unable to disclose in the workplace due to the fear of losing occupational status and prestige. Because work was reported as an important aspect of participants' daily lives, this fear of being open in such an influential sphere of their lives may have serious implications for their well-being in a context of secrecy and fear of discrimination. Furthermore, because the fear of losing legitimacy in their careers was a major barrier preventing participants from being open about their HIV, this prevented any organizational change in occupational settings as this setting was seen as a dangerous place to disclose. By keeping HIV a secret and only disclosing to a few people, participants were able to negotiate their HIV but this strategy did not allow for a change in the social structure, which produced the stigma they had to deal with in the first place. Action occurred through different processes such as involvement in Helping Hand, but a complete overthrow of stigma was not allowed as the social order remained unchanged, perpetuating prevailing social conceptions of HIV.

Perhaps news media and other organizations are more likely to change the existing social order than individuals acting outside the protective and unified context of social groups. The successes of civil rights activists, the gay community, and other social movements suggest that group action can be an effective means for activism and efforts geared towards altering prevailing societal conceptions of HIV. By actively challenging the symbolism surrounding HIV, the meaning of HIV can be changed to correspond to more positive imagery. Also, the use of entertainment such as theater, comedy, music, writing, and other artistic means could help to change the meanings ascribed to HIV. Without the protection of other group members, people can be exposed to stigmatizing societal reactions that entail deep, personal harm.

Indeed, David who displayed a strong activist identity, although he did try to inform communities about HIV, had to pay a heavy price for his activism. A local newspaper covered the story of David informing local communities about HIV. Despite their promises of confidentiality, David's identity was revealed, exposing his HIV status against his consent. After the story came out in the news, David was treated differently by people he had known for years. He lost many friends and felt that the exposure of his HIV status caused people to distance themselves from him and to end their relationships with him. The anticipation of stigma that participants felt was not an unfounded fear, being open about HIV status can expose people to devastating social losses, exclusion, and isolation that require a great deal of inner strength and resilience to endure.

Furthermore, HIV is an illness, which due to sexual contact as a mode of transmission, is closely linked with conceptions of promiscuous and deviant sexual behavior David brought up the roles of religion and culture in defining HIV as a product of immoral or sinful sexual behavior such as homosexual contact and infidelity. Because of the link between HIV and sex, David felt that people with HIV were considered to be "whores" (Sequential Report 8, p. 1). He used the example that even if a man was married, he was seen as getting HIV through his own infidelity. David believed that due to the associations between sex, sin, and HIV, HIV was problematized and kept a secret. HIV was seen as having a perceived moral dimension because of its association with sex. The moral dimension attributed to HIV may account for why participants felt that HIV was a secret to carry but that other illnesses such as cancer were acceptable to disclose to others.

Therefore, the decision to live with HIV as a secret can be tied to the societal judgment of HIV as a proxy for "sinful" and "immoral" sexual behavior. The theme of HIV as a secret was closely connected to moral sentiments attached to HIV for the participants interviewed. HIV was described as a stigmatized social status not only because of other's fear of infection, but to the negative associations of people with HIV as being sexually promiscuous, deviant, sinful, and at fault for their illness. HIV was described as a stigma of the body and of character (Goffman 1963). HIV can be a stigma of the body because it is a physical illness that resides in the body and is able to be transmitted to others. Also, HIV emerged as a stigma of character because the mode of transmission is linked to images of sexual, deviant, and immoral behavior. This may help to explain why reducing fear of transmission is not sufficient in reducing fear of HIV. Reducing the fear of transmission may only decrease stigma of the body, not of character. Dual approaches aimed at changing attitudes towards people with HIV from being seen as sexually and morally deviant could help to reduce stigma of character. Examples of people who break negative stereotypes of HIV can help to expand people's conceptions of HIV. Indeed, some of the cases selected for this analysis were not only selected due to theoretical sampling, but also because they presented unique cases of HIV which challenge prevailing negative stereotypes of people with HIV.

Furthermore, stigma appeared to be an intersectional concept. Gay participants reported that being gay was felt as something "on top of HIV." HIV was a status that was intertwined with other social statuses such as race/ethnicity, age, and sexual orientation. Gay male participants emphasized the importance of maintaining secrecy regarding their sexuality and their HIV status in the workplace. For example, Chris was selective in his HIV disclosure and felt that revealing his HIV status could endanger his career, reputation, and fundamentally alter his intimate relationships:

"I think is the hardest part to tell someone 'No I can't be with you' but not like make a reason why because um because if it would be like someone whose familiar with this whole gay lifestyle everything is ok but like first of all he's Mormon (-) he's completely new to this (-) like I'm the first guy he developed feelings for and on top of that I'm positive so it's already hard as it is I think." [Transcript 3, lines 94-101]

Chris rejected this man because he felt that coping with being new to this gay lifestyle was already difficult enough without having to deal with HIV as he explained:

"He told me like he would even out himself to his family and take me home to meet his parents and all that and that's a lot but on top of that to come out and say 'I know you're dealing with all this and this might be hard but on top of that I'm positive' so I think that would just be a lot you know" [Transcript 3; lines 103-107].

The above excerpt suggests that being both HIV-positive and gay can be especially difficult because being gay was felt to be a controversial status and to have HIV "on top of it" could make life more complicated and difficult despite advances in the gay community. Arthur also discussed the layered dimension of being gay and having HIV:

"I would say coming out open with your sexual behavior (-) sexual preferences (-) is one bad point but it's even worse if you say you're gay and having HIV (-) that comes on top of it (-) the bad seed first people would never accept that (-) the people who only deal with you from your job life (-) not your friends or whatever (-) I expect a friend of mine (--) or my brother when I told him about being gay and then later on about being infected if he can't deal with it then I don't have a brother no more (-) and he just accepted it 'Live your own life (-) you live your life (-) I'll live my life' that's what he said (-) he said 'Ok' he accepted it (-) but in the company would be completely different." [Transcript 4, lines 167-173]

Importantly, Arthur used the same terminology as Chris by describing HIV as something that was "on top of" being gay. Arthur felt that being a gay man with HIV would lead him to not be accepted by others due to conceptions of normality, religion, law, and sin. Arthur elaborated:

"There are people (--) homosexuality is the thing which is abnormal (-) some people say it's like animalistic still (-) And depending on the religion as well (-) religious things as well (-) uh well I had a feeling that I was doing something that was unlawful at that time anyway (-) we still had (--) when I was in my twenties or my teens (-) teen (-) teenager years it was still against the law in Germany (-) so you always had the feeling of doing something (--) put you with guilt (-) put (-) put (-) put a weight on your shoulder like and things have changed in a positive way […] people know I have no problem with that no more (-) earlier (-) like twenty years ago (-) that was different." [Transcript 4, lines 229-240]

Acceptance was important to Arthur. The illegality of homosexuality made Arthur feel that he was doing something unacceptable which he had to conceal and that placed a "weight" and "guilt" upon him. This illustrates how social conceptions of sin and morality can reflect public views of normality, which can be internalized, and in the case of Arthur, may lead to a dissonance and self-questioning linked to his possession of a deviant and even illegal identity. Arthur started his interview by explaining that he has been gay all his life and so here he described a critical moment in his personal history which was rooted in the German historical context of anti-gay laws. Arthur defined himself as gay and in the present no longer felt that he was abnormal or a criminal. However, in the past legal prohibition towards gays made him feel guilty and ashamed of his sexual identity.

Arthur discussed his feelings of guilt and shame and felt that his emotions were linked to what was socially acceptable or legal and hence defined as normal. This discussion by Arthur illustrated how public concerns can transform into a private crisis. Indeed, Scheff (1990) posited that shame is a socialized emotion that emerges based on other's perceptions and our awareness of these evaluations. Because Arthur was aware of the negative views society had of his sexuality this shook his foundations of his view of himself. This awareness contributed to an existential problem of questioning the morality of his sexuality and to a reorientation towards social reality and his relationship to the social world. These emotional struggles were related to societal conceptions of categories such as "gay" or "HIV" being problematized in society and stigmatized.

Arthur felt that he had to hide his sexuality and to maintain his lifestyle and identity in complete secrecy. Secrecy emerged as a perceived necessity in living with socially contested and problematized social statuses. As suggested by Arthur's case, this existential dilemma also highlighted the political nature of stigma. Stigma had the power to problematize categories and social groups, and to also exclude and discriminate. Importantly, the case of Arthur suggests that stigma can also initiate an internal debate that involves self-questioning, guilt, shame, and secrecy. Importantly, Arthur brought up the issue of social change as he explained that attitudes towards gays have changed in a "positive way." He provided the example of his current living situation with his neighbors and how his neighbors knew he was gay and it was not an issue. Arthur felt that now his gayness was not a major issue for him because people's attitudes towards gays have changed. In the past Arthur had to conceal his sexuality and he emphasized the difficulties maintaining this secret. Interestingly, Arthur felt that his sexuality was a source of gossip and that this gossip was especially prominent in the work place. Gossip again emerged as an important aspect of stigma. Reflecting back on his life, Arthur felt that with his experiences since then he would have chosen to live a different life and made a distinction between those whose opinions mattered and less salient social relationships. While Arthur felt if given the choice he would have lived a different life and been more open, it is not clear if would have due to the strong pressure to remain silent he experienced.

Chris also distinguished between those who mattered and those who he felt were not close to him and thus whose opinions were not important. Chris wanted to be seen for whom he felt he truly was a popular, social, and happy person. He did not want to be treated as an outcast or for others to alter their perceptions of him based on his HIV status. Similar to Chris, George was a teacher. George felt that his coworkers may have had some idea that he was gay or had HIV because he was very sick last summer. However, he would not actively go open about his sexual orientation or HIV status because he reported feeling afraid of jeopardizing his career and reputation. Similar to Chris, George reported feeling that parents could become very fearful of him as a teacher if he disclosed his HIV status because he worked with children. George also did not want HIV to become a master status that defined how others view him. George explained that he did not want his students or their parents to know anything about his personal life. George felt that personal and professional life should be separate. George gave an example that some of his teaching colleagues may have known that he was gay but if he would come out people would act differently. George explained that if people knew he was gay others would attribute all his actions as being due to his sexual orientation and his sexuality would become a master status and shape how others defined his behavior. Being gay and having HIV can be seen as the intersection of two deviant and problematized social statuses, which can create a unique set of challenges for people with HIV who are gay. The intersection of HIV stigma with other social statuses suggests that stigma is an intersectional concept that cannot be examined in a social vacuum.

In addition, there may be no need for a debate of the terms discrimination versus stigma because both are part of a process. Discrimination is the external treatment while stigma is the relation of a deviant status to negative stereotypes. The term experienced or enacted stigma can be seen as including discrimination and the experience of an awareness of stigma. Stigma can be seen as an experience and to understand stigma it is important to understand both the experience of discrimination (acts by others to exclude and marginalize) as well as how stigma (being linked with a marginalized status) is experienced. Because stigma is a process-based concept, with numerous secondary processes, conceptualizing stigma as dynamic, intersectional, and process-based and as rooted in history, social context, and power dynamics allows for an elaboration of the concept of stigma as encouraged by prior researchers who have argued for an extension of the concept of stigma (Link and Phelan 2001; Parker and Aggleton 2003). Furthermore, because stigma involves power dynamics research on stigma should also focus on agency and how people in a context of adversity and marginalization act to change their life circumstances and to potentially reclaim power and legitimacy. The current analysis, by examining action, resources such as social support, and stigma simultaneously, helps to elaborate the interrelations between these phenomena, thus further developing the process-based conceptualization of stigma.

Importantly, stigma was a major concern for PLWHA in both Frankfurt and Miami. Similar to the Frankfurt sample, participants also reported a fear of being seen using HIV services due to an anticipation of stigma. Even those who eventually decided to go public with their HIV status reflected on the difficulty of the decision to be open about their HIV status. Being involved in support groups and talking with others of different sexualities and backgrounds about HIV helped to reduce the fear of stigma and helped participants to feel connected to others. This also emphasized the intersection of being gay and of having HIV because connecting to others who had HIV and who had different sexualities was described as important in coming to terms with the fear of stigma. Conceptions of sin related to sexuality, sexual practices, and drug use can further problematize HIV stigma. This is similar to the discussion in the Frankfurt sample of being gay as something that was layered on top of HIV stigma. Similar to the Frankfurt sample, the intersectionality of HIV stigma with stigma related to sexuality was discussed among interviewees in Miami. Gay participants discussed how being gay was tied to their experiences with HIV. Experiences of stigma due to being gay could heighten fears and anticipation of HIV stigma. Working out feelings of stigma due to sexuality or other statuses helped participants to reduce their fears of HIV stigma. However, others discussed anticipation of stigma in the context of intimate relationships as an ongoing struggle and this is discussed below.

3.9.6.2   Stigma, Appearance, and Problems in Intimate Partnerships

Interestingly, the issue of appearance in avoiding stigma and gaining a sense of normalcy was emphasized. The use of cosmetic procedures to correct skin damage due to lipodystrophy was described as allowing participants to look healthy and avoid stigma. This suggests that instead of dismissing the importance of physical appearance, approaches to reduce the pain of stigma could involve making cosmetic, restorative procedures available to those who experience disfigurements marking them as different. Similar to the Frankfurt sample, appearance was an aspect of self-presentation that was negotiated to prevent stigma. Problems with adjusting to marks on their appearance from illness were described as alienating and emotionally distressful. Being able to hide the mark of HIV and to regain a positive self-image was related to being treated in a more socially acceptable manner. Minor cosmetic procedures appeared to make participants feel more comfortable interacting with others and to improve their life conditions. Issues of weight loss and appearance related to HIV were discussed in both samples. Extreme thinness and other physical characteristics considered a negative or unhealthy change in appearance made participants in both samples feel exposed, marked as sick, and contributed to their withdrawing from others. Therefore, being able to positively enhance appearance was a means of regaining control over the visibility of HIV and to maintain a positive self-image. The importance of physical appearance and the body thus should not be neglected in studies of stigma. Indeed, the importance of presentation of self and of appearance and the body in social interaction have been emphasized in prior research (Goffman 1959; Schütz 1962). For PLWHA who are contending with a socially contested and discredited status, appearance can be a means of negotiating interaction to regain a sense of normalcy and social acceptance.

Although appearance was important, it served to only hide stigma from other's evaluations and did not act to combat stigma in an active and open way because stigma remained in the shadows behind the external world of social performance and interaction. For people with HIV, the dramaturgical aspects of social life were pronounced. Similar to the participants in Frankfurt who reported living a double life or described their HIV as a secret, participants in Miami felt they had to engage in a performance and to present themselves in a socially acceptable way while acting on stage in the HIV-negative world. While participants could choose to hide their HIV if their appearance was not affected by illness, the stigma could still be revealed in social interaction and reacted to in socially rejecting ways upon disclosure. The awareness that revealing HIV status could fundamentally alter social relationships and interaction was a consideration that participants in both samples emphasized.

Although participants could hide their HIV status behind their appearance, not disclosing was described as stressful and limiting the openness and intimacy of relationships. Rejection in romance was a recurrent theme for participants in both samples and was a major ongoing concern. Rejection was related to feeling unwanted and feared, and violated prior conceptions of the self as socially accepted and sexually desirable. Problems in establishing intimate relationships were ongoing for participants and they repeatedly emphasized problems in dating and feeling limited in the types of partners they could have. The constant rejection and perceived lowering of standards in dating were described as extremely painful. Difficulties in dating and finding love were important to participants in both samples and HIV was felt as a barrier to establishing intimate relationships and to the eventual formation of a family, thus potentially blocking membership in a socially "normal" institution, the family. For those who had romantic partners or children, their relationships with their families were described as extremely important to their well-being. This suggests that having information about ways to engage in sexual behavior and to have children could greatly expand the possibilities for life chances that PLWHA perceive.

Importantly, even those with education about HIV were described as being stigmatizing towards people with HIV. This suggests that information about modes of HIV transmission was not sufficient in reducing this deep fear of infection and perhaps a deeper fear of mortality. Indeed, prior research on the effectiveness of anti-stigma interventions for HIV suggests that information alone is not enough to reduce stigma and that HIV may represent a deeper threat to mortality and normality that is not reduced with information about HIV alone (Brown et al. 2003). Some examples of stigmatizing behaviors experienced by interviewees included having others refuse to eat food prepared by participants, partners steaming out their showers, and the loss of professional careers.

3.9.6.3   Stigma Proliferation

Another dimension of stigma that emerged in the analysis was stigma proliferation also known as secondary stigma or "courtesy stigma" (Goffman 1963). Participants reported anticipating that their loved ones would also be stigmatized if they were to disclose their HIV status. Prior research has identified secondary stigma as a phenomena that occurs internationally with studies documenting secondary stigma in Asia, Africa, and other countries (Salter et al. 2010; Ogunmefun et al. 2011; Herek 1996). Sarah explained:

> "As for stigma (-) well that was (--) well of course it was the (-) the (-) the mhhh anxiety or (-) or the this waiting the negative stigma (-) something like that (-) which made me to keep it for myself (-) and I (-) and I thought of the children (-) I was thinking of the children that they would be stigmatized and that I wanted to avoid in any case (-) it could have happened in those days (-) I mean knowing in the kindergarten 'Oh the mother is HIV-positive?' you couldn't (-) you couldn't have said they would have maybe somehow have been (--) not really excluded uh concretely but you know (-) they could (-) they could have noticed it (-) and so I wanted to spare them never told anybody." [Transcript 5, lines 61-72]

Sarah wanted to "spare" her sons from being stigmatized and she framed this in the context of how an awareness of her HIV status in her children's educational sphere of life could have negatively impacted her children. Her decision to not disclose was grounded in her concern of the potential outreaching effects of HIV stigma to her family. This indicated that in Sarah's case, a proliferation of stigma involved stigma of the person who possessed the delegitimized and problematized status of HIV and was so powerful that this stigma had the potential to undermine intimate others' social status even at a very young age. However, because Sarah did not disclose it was not clear if this would have actually occurred or if this would have only remained an anticipation of secondary stigma.

Nancy also discussed not wanting to expose her sons to her life with HIV in order to protect them. Also, Nancy chose to not disclose to her mother. When Nancy was diagnosed the first person she thought of was her mother she explained:

> "How could I tell her this? 'If I tell her this is she strong enough to handle it?' but I told myself 'No after today my mother doesn't know about it'." (Sequential Report 6, p. 2)

Even though Nancy's mother was worried because she was getting sick, Nancy never told her about her HIV. Nancy did not tell her mother because she felt that she was everything to her mother, and felt that as the eldest child of her mother they shared a deep relationship. Nancy was afraid of losing her mother and her mother was afraid of losing Nancy. They shared a concern for each other's health and Nancy felt it was very difficult to live with HIV because she could not tell her mother who was the person closest to her. For Nancy, her best friend was her mother. Paradoxically, their closeness prevented her disclosure. Nancy was always looking for a way to tell her mother. Her mother had recently visited her and Nancy tried to tell her mother but she could not because she was concerned for her mother's health as she explained that while she felt it was wrong to not tell her at the same time she was scared that the news would be very detrimental to her mother's health.

Nancy was also concerned with the possibility of her children being stigmatized and of worrying her mother to literal sickness. Keeping HIV a secret allowed Nancy to protect her loved ones but prevented her from being able to seek support from those closest to her. Nancy also told that she and her ex-husband defined HIV as a private family problem because if they were to tell others, people may have been afraid of both of them. Nancy's boyfriend also preferred to keep this to himself and so her HIV remained between them.

3.9.6.4   Stigma Experienced

Experiences of stigma were often described in tandem with a description of bodily states, namely of extreme thinness due to weight loss. Appearance was reported as key to experienced stigma. Being extremely thin, a type of thinness seen as not natural and as being associated with AIDS, served as a marker of HIV status. Extreme thinness or wasting was associated by others with AIDS and HIV was in turn associated with AIDS. Appearance was an important marker of HIV status because HIV was a stigma that participants felt could be hidden. For example, although Walter felt that there were certain cases where someone could be identified as having HIV, he and others described HIV as a status that could be hidden. Group membership was not easily visible and the "marks" of HIV were ambiguous. Some participants reported experiencing drastic weight loss due to their HIV, which was described as marking them as sick and as contributing to feelings of emotional distress that were so severe that they withdrew from their social surroundings. Indeed, when asked what the difference was between someone who was stigmatized and who was not stigmatized due to HIV, Chris responded that appearance was the distinguishing factor. Chris emphasized appearance as he provided the following example:

> "As long as you're cute looking (-) or as long as people find you attractive in some way or you fit into um the picture somehow you're ok (-) but as soon as you don't fit in the picture by your looks people will treat you different yeah (--) that's just how I see it and what I experience and the good thing is I worked at a sex shop for five years (-) at a gay sex shop also and um back then I was young (-) and um I saw people walk in there and I could automatically (-) I was like

'yeah he's probably sick (-) he probably has HIV' because they were really skinny and their cheek bones were like (-) you could tell and when I came here to the clinic and he told me how the people look who are positive or aren't positive fifteen (-) twenty years ago and explained or described how they look I automatically thought 'yeah'(-) whenever I thought this person or that person may have it cause they look exactly the way he described it (-) so I was the one to say 'uh no (-) I'll judge these people just cause of their looks' and avoid talking to them (-) but if someone cute came in I'd look at him like 'oh that's a cute guy' and didn't even waste a thought of 'yeah he could be positive'." [Transcript 3, lines 363-381]

When Chris used to work at a gay sex shop he would evaluate people and judge them based on their appearance. Specifically, those who were extremely thin with sunken cheek bones were regarded as having HIV. Chris admitted to judging and avoiding people based upon their appearance. Before being diagnosed with HIV, Chris had a desire for social distance from those he thought may have HIV. However, if someone came who Chris considered to be attractive the possibility of that person having HIV did not even cross his mind. Extreme thinness served as a symbolic marker of HIV status which profoundly shaped social interaction. Social interaction was recognized as fluid, temporal, and subject to change. Therefore, social interaction was especially dangerous for participants because their identities were surrounded by negative symbolism. It has been suggested that action, performance, and appearance are fundamentally related:

"Action and appearance relate to performance as conditions that define a person's perception of the purpose as well as to anticipated consequences of his or her performance." (Corbin and Strauss 1988, p. 56-57)

Following this conceptualization of action as intimately tied to symbolic meanings ascribed to bodily states, which can have consequences for the mode of representation of actors, thinness is a factor which can contextualize experience. A critical point made by Strauss was that having an experience can have a lasting effect by changing identity and that a change in identity can then shape future interaction (Strauss 1993). The ongoing interaction between undergoing the experience of stigma, identity, and social interaction emerged in the narratives.

Furthermore, if stigma can be conceptualized as involving a mark (Jones et al. 1984) that links someone to a deviant status, then the ambiguity of HIV status brings our attention to the issue of the construction of the mark of HIV. The mark was negotiated and contested by those who carried it but stigma was more than a mark, it involved numerous secondary processes that occurred at different levels of social reality as suggested by other stigma researchers (see Link and Phelan 2001; Parker and Aggleton 2003). Stigma was rooted, as Link and Phelan

(2001) argued, in power and resources but also emerged in relations to self and others. This indicates that an examination of self-views and views of others (with and without HIV) are important aspects of stigma. For example, Rachel experienced stigmatizing reactions from others and yet appeared to be more accepting of her illness than Walter. Rachel experienced stigma in both her native and host countries. Before Rachel's arrival in Germany she explained that:

> "I was not eating (-) I had no appetite so I only think 'I'm going to die (-) I'm going to die' and when the people look at you they say 'look at this one she's sick' so instead of going out I just remained in the house (-) lie down and stay there I didn't go anywhere (-) yeah so I was very happy to leave that place." [Transcript 2, lines 81-88]

Rachel used emphasis when describing her physical appearance at this time using the term "small." Rachel described that her appearance was an important factor that shaped how people treated her and that people would look at her and see how thin she was and label her as being sick. Because of how others looked at her Rachel did not want to go out, avoided people, and stayed at home. Therefore, her fears of being stigmatized lead her to socially isolate herself. Experienced stigma can contribute to anticipation of more stigma, thus leading to strategies to avoid others such as social isolation.

Rachel experienced more stigma during her stay in Eastern Germany, a time during which she was extremely ill and thin. Rachel described a transitional period when she traveled between two cities and also emphasized how people from her own native country gossiped about her. Again, the importance of Rachel's physical appearance in shaping how others perceived her was emphasized. Rachel's "smallness" and "thinness" were cues to others that Rachel was not "normal" but was sick even though Rachel told no one about her HIV status. Rachel's thinness provided others with visual cues which exposed her illness and made it visible against her will to others. This experience demonstrates the profound alienation that people can experience when their HIV status is visible to others in a context where it has not yet been determined to be safe or in one's best interest to disclose. Verbal stigma in the form of gossip took away Rachel's power to choose the conditions of her HIV-disclosure and forced her into uncomfortable social interactions and an unwanted social status. The biographical context of being in a new country and the bodily state of thinness shaped her experience of stigma and her interactions with others. Rachel emphasized how others would gossip about her and her illness. People displayed a desire for social distance by not wanting to even sit near her and began to maliciously gossip about Rachel's health. Rachel recalled this clearly and described how people were inquiring about her health and how Rachel told no one about HIV but the women around her still talked about her health and spread hurtful rumors. Alone in a new country, she felt she could not even trust or rely on people from her own country. Also, the reaction of the mother of Rachel's boyfriend to her HIV was negative and the mother did not "accept" her HIV. This lack of acceptance was very harmful to Rachel as she recalled:

> "She hates me (-) so that's how I feel she doesn't like me and when she talks sometimes she says 'ah you give me the children' uh when I had when I first had my first born she ah took the child away (-) and when I ask her 'why do you take my child away?' she say 'yeah that child has to be used to me because your time is not long' yeah (-) that's what she she say." [Transcript 2, lines 250-255]

Rachel was being treated as if she was already dead by someone who did not understand that Rachel was able to live with HIV and that HIV was no longer a death sentence. This also suggests that stigma can be disruptive in family relations and should be further examined in familial context. It is possible that in a context of familial conflict children of people living with HIV could be at an increased risk of exposure to witnessing the abuse of their parents and this could have long-term effects on their emotional well-being. Rachel described how she and her boyfriend had to live with this woman:

> "I could not sleep (-) I and when I sleep I just thinking about the lady yeah (-) and (--) after I was having um (-) headache (-) everyday (-) when I came here to doctor and tell them I have headache and they told me I have high blood pressure (-) yeah (-) and to still now I am still taking this medication medicine for high blood pressure (-) if it was not for this woman I wouldn't have (-) maybe (-) I wouldn't have that." [Transcript 2, lines 257-271]

Rachel still had to take medication for her high blood pressure and felt that if it had not been for this experience she would not have problems with her high blood pressure. Rachel's feelings of stress due to feeling rejected and hated affected her health and she experienced sleep disruptions, stress, and headaches. Rachel's account was illustrative because it demonstrated that when living in a social context of powerlessness and rejection (i.e. powerlessness due to lack of privacy and not having her own home and rejection due to feeling unaccepted and hated) stress can negatively impact health and this decline in health can be long-lasting even after the stress of being in such an environment has been removed from someone's life.

These negative consequences of stigma can then be viewed as secondary processes which can affect health and access to resources. The case of Rachel clearly demonstrates a secondary process or consequence of stigma where being stigmatized by her boyfriend's mother lead her to feel stressed, and this stress in turn affected her physical health as manifested by her development of high blood pressure. The processes of being rejected or experiencing social distance can lead to a decision to withdraw from others, serving to further isolate people with HIV. Isolation can then in turn further limit access to social and economic resources. Indeed, prior research demonstrates that stigma can limit access to resources and this can damage health (Link and Phelan 2006; Link et al. 1997). Therefore, it is critical to examine stigma, stress, and health and to ground such an analysis in experience so that these processes can be viewed in biographical context. Similar to the case of Walter, Rachel lived a secret life. She did not trust those "on the outside" to keep her secret of HIV. Rachel discussed the time she was in East Germany:

> "Nobody (-) I told nobody that I'm sick I never told someone that I'm sick the only person that I told was my mom but they (-) the people they just look at you they see you are not healthy enough (-) you are thin (-) you don't look like the others. Then they have this imaginations and they (-) this person (--) knows just about that and tells the other and then it goes further." [Transcript 2, lines 182-190]

The issue of appearance in shaping other's conceptions of someone as healthy or "normal" as opposed to sick or "deviant" was emphasized in her interview. Rachel told no one about her HIV status but based on physical marks such as her weight, others began to judge that Rachel was too thin and not like "the others" and from these ideas, rumors began to spread. This information diffused across social networks as Rachel felt powerless to stop it. Although Walter did not discuss having experienced any drastic weight loss or having experienced people spreading rumors about him, Rachel and Walter both were aware how information could be spread through social networks and how people without HIV could treat them in a social discriminatory way by isolating and rejecting them. Fear of rejection and a desire to not have a reputation as someone who was sick was emphasized. Also, the fear of rejection and desire to not possess a de-legitimatized identity prevented participants from trusting other people and from disclosing their HIV status.

Nancy reported experiencing stigma while seeking care at the dentist. When Nancy told the dentist she had HIV, the staff told her they would give her a later appointment which Nancy perceived as being another way of saying "if you are positive you don't belong here" (Sequential Report 6, p. 6). Nancy heard similar stories from other patients at the clinic who told her about being stigmatized while seeking medical care. Another example of experiencing stigma in a medical setting was reported by David who sought treatment for back pain. David disclosed his HIV status to the doctor examining his back and described how the doctor then rushed through his examination and did not find anything abnormal. However, David then sought treatment from another doctor who did a more thorough examination and found a tumor that needed to be removed. This demonstrates how poor medical treatment can result from stigma and can thus be another secondary process through which stigma can affect health. Furthermore, because doctors have high educational attainment and are knowledgeable about HIV transmission, this suggests that education and information about HIV transmission were not enough to reduce fear of HIV. This has implications for anti-stigma movements geared at changing public conceptions of HIV by providing education about HIV transmission. Such efforts may therefore benefit from more initiatives such as reducing blame for HIV and redefining HIV from an issue related to drug addiction, sex, sin, and immorality to a health issue that can affect a broad range of people. Such initiatives could also be directed towards health professionals. Discussions of experiencing social distance or physical stigma also emerged in the analysis. Before joining Helping Hand, similar to Walter, Rachel did not talk to the other patients there. I probed further into how Rachel was treated before and she elaborated on how experiencing social distance hurt her feelings and the pain of having people taking care to avoid even sitting next to her. I probed into how this made her feel and she responded that it made her feel sad and anxious.

At this point in her interview she sighed, suggesting that this was a heavy topic to discuss and implying the emotional burden of these experiences of rejection. Rachel reacted to people who treated her badly by avoiding them. She felt self-conscious that others would look at her and think that she was sick so she avoided being around people. Therefore, Rachel's strategy prior to joining Helping Hand was to avoid others and avoidance of others allowed her to not have to have to explain her appearance. Other interviewees also reported not wanting to have to answer questions and a preference for secrecy to avoid explanations of their health status. Having to explain one's life situation and to deal with questions was reported as stressful. Deviance, by definition, is an exception from the norm, and exceptions from the norm often require explanation because of the questions such exceptions incite. Therefore, those with HIV were faced with the issue of having to deal with numerous questions about themselves.

The unspoken questions regarding Rachel's health overwhelmed her and she did not want to have to confront these inquiries and instead chose to withdraw from others. Appearance and privacy may therefore shape the visibility of HIV, which suggests that circumstances that allow people with HIV to have control over their appearance and privacy may reduce feelings of visibility and discomfort. Indeed, Rachel discussed how her initial stay in Germany was characterized by a lack of privacy as she lived in a house for asylum seekers. Rachel's personal history of immigrating to Germany was an important experience contextualizing her life with HIV. Immigration can intersect with experiences of HIV and stigma. For example, Rachel, Nancy, and Walter were not native to Germany and their stories involved a discussion of being processed through a new system while in Germany. Experiences in the immigration system and the importance of participants' countries of origin emerged as important themes that contextualized their experience of HIV and shaped their view of medical treatment. This is further emphasized the importance of examining how stigma was experienced in comparative perspective.

Stigma by one family member can transform the family dynamic into a situation where the family becomes divided. Experiences of stigma in the family were discussed in the Miami data. Vivid descriptions of being ostracized by family members and the conflicts between family members taking sides emerged as a problematic aspect of living with HIV. In order to ensure confidentiality the details of these conflicts could not be reported. However, there were troubling stories of participants feeling that they were defending their lives and feeling deeply hurt by the need to convince family members that they were not deadly "monsters" or "weapons." The stigma of HIV fundamentally altered relationships with family members in a profoundly negative and isolating manner. This suggests that in response to stigma, people have to work to challenge the negative stereotypes others link to their HIV status and to redefine the social meanings others are applying to them in the most intimate parts of their lives. Also, experiencing stigma can damage self-worth and become internalized. Emotional work was described as integral to self-acceptance and love of self in the face of HIV stigma. Experiencing stigma was an emotional trauma and the feeling that if people could survive the emotional trauma of HIV then they could live with the HIV was emphasized. Importantly, it was felt that the people who stigmatize PLWHA that were killing people with HIV, emphasizing the pain and suffering of experiencing stigma. Participants negotiated intersecting trajectories of suffering where they had to contend with the suffering of the illness itself and its threat to existential meaning. They also had to negotiate the suffering of stigma and the awareness that even if their stigma was hidden, upon disclosure they could risk losing their social standing and relationships. The feeling that HIV stigma was more deadly and harmful than HIV itself was discussed in both samples, which emphasized the deep suffering of stigma. This demonstrates the importance of studying stigma when focusing on the experience of living with HIV. A benefit of this qualitative analysis was that it enabled the examination of HIV diagnosis, disclosure, and the ways that people were empowered to work at improving their lives in relation to HIV stigma and within the context of their lives. Anticipating and experiencing stigma emerged as an integral part of living with HIV and created a context of fear, isolation, and exclusion in participants' life worlds in both samples. The discussion of spirituality suggested that when dealing with HIV and HIV-stigma, people go through complex processes of meaning making that involved a deep interconnection of beliefs regarding humanity, the spiritual, truth, and their self-views.

The distinction of taking sides relates to the conception of a split in social reality. Similar to the participants in the Frankfurt sample, participants in Miami had to contend with a split in social reality due to a division in group membership in the HIV-negative and positive communities and had to negotiate a contested and feared status, which suggested a need for protection and understanding. This was especially hurtful because it happened within the context of romantic relationships and family.

An important emergent finding was that for some participants experiencing stigma motivated activism. Stigma was felt as pushing participants to the limits of their endurance and giving them a sense of mission. The conviction that there was work to be done in order to eliminate stigma and to raise awareness that people with HIV were not to be feared was expressed. Experiences of stigma in some cases contributed to feelings of both anger and assertiveness and to a strengthening of conviction. There was a sense of injustice towards exclusion others placed on people with HIV. If even their families could not trust them how could they convince others that they were not contagious weapons? It was repeatedly emphasized that information about the route of infection was not enough to reduce stigma. Because information about HIV was not sufficient to reduce stigma there appeared to be deeply rooted emotional aspects to stigmatizing attitudes and behaviors. HIV seemed to present a perceived existential threat to mortality and reality among those without HIV. This fear served to denigrate people with HIV to a subhuman status where they were seen as a means to HIV infection and thus treated as deadly. This is consistent with the social constructionist view that death and the imagery surrounding illness can be threatening and a source of existential terror of a loss of meaning and existence (Berger and Luckmann 1966)

Therefore, understanding the personal histories of both those stigmatizing and those experiencing stigmatization is important in developing approaches to reduce stigma and to understand its etiology. Discussions of stigma were present even among those who initially reported they had not actually experienced stigma because they had not disclosed in the Frankfurt sample. Participants in Frankfurt did not disclose because they had an anticipation and fear of stigma. Also, those who disclosed to a few close people also reported rejecting, socially distancing reactions.

Interestingly, in the Miami sample there were descriptions of having visions. One such vision involved the government where one participant envisioned the president of the United States telling them that they did not "count" and that the government wrote off people with HIV. This perceived communication with the government symbolized feelings of marginalization within the context of American government and the broader political structure. In response to feeling written off and dismissed in society a participant in the Miami sample adapted create a momentum of action in order to create and to produce something meaningful out of the conventional workforce. The response of innovation and creative production outside the bounds of conventionality helped to not only maintain personal drive and inspiration but to work to create awareness about HIV and to facilitate social change. Involvement in creative work was used as a means of personal expression and HIV-activism. However, creative pursuits were not easy because of limited opportunities and setbacks due to disclosing HIV status and the ensuing discrimination. In the face of adversity, persistence was felt to be a key factor in developing access to opportunities. Therefore, innovation and persistence emerged as important aspects of the biographical work needed to create opportunities despite being excluded. Navigating a new world outside the bounds of normality was critical in adapting to HIV and overcoming stigma.

Holidays were cultural symbols of normality and were observed to maintain a sense of coherence despite the stigma of HIV. Holidays, having families, maintaining friendships and work, and being a part of society were important to participants in both samples. Striving for a sense of normality when faced with a new life situation characterized by threats to morality, problems in negotiating chronic illness, and stigma was a means of regaining control and coherence to seemingly chaotic life change. HIV was a major life-changing event that participants had to navigate and to overcome by working to regain a sense of coherence and meaning in their lives. HIV-stigma rendered the experience of HIV even more stressful, jeopardizing intimate relationships with romantic partners and family, friendships, and careers. A recurrent theme among both samples was the relationship of HIV-stigma to professional standing and career opportunities. HIV-stigma limited life chances of employment among the Miami sample and among the Frankfurt sample the fear of stigma in the workplace prevented disclosure.

The interplay between the world of work and occupational spheres with the world of HIV and HIV stigma was a fundamental aspect of living with HIV. Stigma in occupational settings not only limited opportunities for work and jeopardized professional reputations and standings, but also created a restrictive social context which contributed to less openness about HIV. Being open about HIV and working to create opportunities in the resulting "vacuum" of social rejection required a strong will and commitment to persevere. The survivor mentality of relentless persistence was a valuable tool in combating stigma. Descriptions of being relentless and being a "workaholic" were involved in discussions of HIV-activism. This persistence was critical when negotiating stigma and working to create personal and social change in a context where participants paid the heavy price of their professional careers and closest relationships. HIV-activism was framed as a decision between helping others and creating social change versus financial stability. Financial concerns were a recurrent theme and so the tension between the need for financial stability and losing professional opportunities had a profound impact on personal and professional lives.

HIV-stigma problematized multiple aspects of life experience. With the awareness that revealing HIV to others could fundamentally alter even the most taken for granted relationships, reality and truth became contested. When making sense of HIV, participants struggled with epistemological debates regarding the nature of reality and truth. A striking similarity between some participants in both samples was their view of reality being beneath the surface. Just as HIV could be concealed, the truth of "normal interaction" could also be hidden. Some participants knocked on the tables in front of them when they discussed their conceptions of reality and truth and felt that there was more to reality than what was on the surface or manifested in the external world. Both luck and conspiring governmental powers were forces felt as beyond their immediate control but the choice of representation of the loss of control was related to the cultural context of participants' lives.

For example, Walter was African American and adhered to Islam and he drew on his awareness of racism and distrust of the government when debating the nature of reality. Conceptions of the nature of reality were related to views of the nature of their HIV, of its cause, purpose, and the role it played in their lives. Views of reality, society, the self, and HIV were intricately intertwined. In order to understand how HIV was experienced and HIV-stigma was lived with, understanding these beliefs and views were pivotal. HIV presented a threat to mortality, self-view, and sense of belonging, thus creating an existential dilemma where participants had to draw on their pre-existing notions of reality, themselves, and society that were rooted in their biographies. Participants contextualized existing schemes of meaning within frames of reference grounded in the local and structural contexts of their lives. This ongoing process of meaning making was a means of negotiating threat and of doing biographical work to recast HIV with new meaning and to reintegrate their identities into a coherent whole.

Participants in both samples emphasized the importance of truth. Some realized a common human interest and felt that everyone desired to have greatness, life was a journey, others were not to be judged, and viewed the Bible as a means to truth. Despite struggle with the stigmatizing religious doctrines and moral discourse of the Bible coming to terms with struggles related to conceptions of sin helped in the finding of and found meaning in its stories. The idea of a common human journey was present in both samples. For example, Walter was Muslim and felt that all of humanity shared a path despite his sense of injustice at his HIV. Identifying with humanity and its desires and struggles was related to establishing a sense of belonging despite mistreatment and alienation. In the Miami sample, self-definitions of the self as spiritual and the desire to embrace religion and to be loving despite the felt chaos of the world was an aspect of biographical work aimed at unconditional love.

Working to reconcile spiritual struggles was related to religious conflicts and reintegrating HIV into biography in a coherent way, which provided a sense of purpose and meaning, was related to acceptance. Importantly, this was not a static state of being. The maintenance of a loving and compassionate view of humanity required constant negotiation and was an ongoing achievement. Compassion was worked at continuously to contend with marginalization and conflict and to enhance feelings of acceptance. Compassion was related to acceptance of HIV and could explain why those who had accepted HIV used their creative outlets to discuss HIV, whereas Walter who was in denial would not write about HIV. When struggling with a new life in a foreign and threatening social terrain of illness and social rejection, stigma can render the experience of adaptation to the new world of HIV as especially problematic. HIV stigma was a barrier to social integration and limited possibilities of social acceptance and meaningful interaction and relationships with others. However, through multiple processes, participants worked to overcome the barrier of stigma and to lead productive, meaningful lives. Importantly, this work was continual and stigma was a constant barrier that required continuous effort over time to negotiate.

Religious stigma was emphasized in the Miami sample. HIV was compared to leprosy and because God did not fear lepers and accepted them, it was felt that HIV should also be accepted as a disease and not feared by the church. Also, having a past lifestyle of drug use and risky sexual behavior was felt as a barrier to religious involvement because of feelings of not being accepted by others. In response to this feeling of stigma, one participant described using their HIV as "weapon" to combat stigma. However, over time the stigma of HIV was too overwhelming and contributed to a withdrawal of attempts to combat stigma. There were attempts by participants to start HIV support groups in the religious settings but these were unsuccessful because of feeling shunned away by the religious community. It was felt that there were others who were sick in religious institutions that could have benefited from a support group but were too scared to reveal their status and instead turned to their families for support. There were feelings of exclusion even by members of the religious groups that were sick and efforts to raise awareness of HIV in religious settings were discouraged by the unresponsive and fearful reactions of others.

Similar to the Frankfurt sample, verbal stigma emerged as an important concern. Perhaps due to the structure of the Miami interviews, which included questions regarding religion, verbal stigma or gossip was discussed in the Miami sample in relation to religious institutions. Participants discussed fears and experiences of gossip and verbal stigma and because the religious settings were places where they felt vulnerable, visible, and judged by others. This anticipation of stigma could have prevented engagement in religion that could have helped them to work on issues of self-worth, relationships with self and with the spiritual, and ties to the community. This also prevented people with HIV from feeling comfortable enough to disclose their status or to speak about the issue of HIV in religious institutions, which prevented them from accessing a potentially useful social resource that could be utilized to enhance awareness of HIV, financial and emotional support, and provide a social space for support and discourse about HIV with both HIV-negative and HIV-positive people. Indeed, discourse with HIV-negative people was emphasized as being important because it prevented isolation and facilitated personal growth by allowing for interaction with a diverse group of people.

Experiences of mistrust and alienation in a religious context emerged in the interviews as being related to views of the self, others, and God. Also, it is important to consider the overall context of life experiences as they unfold in the institutional domain of religion. For example, some participants experienced abuse in their youth by religious figures. Early childhood experiences of sexual victimization by religious figures had a profound and lasting impact on their views of religion, suggesting that in order to understand how people living with HIV construct their meanings of the spiritual and of religion it is critical to study their biographies as lifelong processes.

In the establishment of a personal sense of the spiritual in the context of stigmatizing religious doctrine, participants had to "face" their HIV and this involved accepting and loving the self, an attunement with the universe, and conceptualizing the universe as a guide. The yearning for a sense of belonging in the face of alienation and isolation was pronounced. By accepting other people's limitations and having a sense of the possibility for the potential for positive change feelings of loneliness and disconnection were overcome. For those with lifestyles and identities that involved being gay, sexually promiscuous, or drug use seeking comfort in religious books and institutions was problematic because often these religious doctrines emphasized sin, damnation, punishment, and blamed their problems on character defects. Religious doctrines were related to conceptions of sin that stained their character corresponding to Goffman's (1963) concept of stigma as a blemish of character. Moral sentiments can serve to blame people with HIV by attributing the cause of their illness to some perceived internal flaw of character. Negative stereotypes of sexuality and HIV status contributed to participants feeling that religion could not help them because of its conceptions of sin. Therefore, the development of a meaningful and personal relationship with the spiritual in accordance with participants' moral sentiments, lifestyles, and beliefs was important in biographical adjustment to HIV.

Reading and integrating other approaches to meaning making helped in the development of hope, the overcoming of fear of religion, and the redefining of personal relationships with God. Before making meaningful connections that integrated identity and moral discourse, participants often internalized stigma. Internalization of stigma was related to feelings of worthlessness. Learning to love the self and others was described as helping participants to move away from resentment and to develop empathy, compassion, and a sense of belonging. Sense of belonging and stigma appeared to have a dynamic relationship where stigma prevented a sense of belonging but a sense of belonging helped to reduce stigma. Developing spirituality helped in the resolution of problems involving sexual stigma, HIV-stigma, and religious conflict. Resolving religious and moral conflicts opened participants to spiritual sources of support and provided them with a sense of belonging to humanity and the spiritual.

The importance of meaning making and the development of a personal relationship with the spiritual emerged as important aspects of the development of a sense of belonging and coping with stigma. Experiences of stigma were deeply personal and embedded in moral discourse surrounding participants' life conditions and social positions. By grounding experiences of stigma and illness in biographical experience, the context-bound and complex processes of biographical work aimed at overcoming trajectories of suffering were identified. When studying HIV and other health conditions, we can produce meaningful theoretical insights by utilizing a comparative biographical approach. Stigma was discussed in both samples suggesting that stigma is a cross-cultural and trans-continental phenomenon for PLWHA. Structural conditions such as social policies related to health care, immigration, and economic resources emerged as import-ant contextual concerns within which the experiences of stigma and coping with HIV were embedded.

3.10   Part 4: Structural Aspects of Negotiating HIV

3.10.1   Migration as Context and Biographical Position

Experiences of stigma must be grounded in their social context in order to be more fully understood. One benefit of conducting these interviews at a clinic in an international, major metropolitan area of Germany was access to interview participants who came from a range of cultural and national backgrounds. This allowed for an examination of how migration processes were related to stigma experiences. Stigma was discussed by both native Germans and migrants. However, the context of stigma provided grounding for their description of these stigma experiences.

As illustrated in the case of Rachel, who upon her arrival in Germany was forced to go to East Germany far away from her mother and to stay in another house for asylum seekers, political arrangements in the form of immigration law can shape the spatial context of daily life and have a profound impact on experiences of stigma. Rachel described a feeling of being processed by the German immigration system against her will as she explained her feelings of being "taken" to Eastern Germany. This description was similar to Walter's feelings of "being instructed" to receive medical treatment. Both used processing terms when describing their procedural experiences with the German immigration and health care systems, respectively. Perhaps this indicates their feelings of resistance and frustration when faced with a new and foreign institutionalized system. Migration experiences contextualized experiences of stigma. The conceptualization of country of origin as a condition that contextualizes the migration process, its experiences, and within which stigma is lived through, follows the guidance of Strauss (1993) to use a framework of a "conditional matrix" when analyzing biography (Corbin and Strauss 2007). Using the analytical tool of a conditional matrix can provide ways of conceptualizing and identifying conditions that have an influence on emergent phenomenon.

Accordingly, country of origin appeared to be a contextual condition that shaped experiences in relation to migration, stigma, and coping. The only participant interviewed in Germany who was from the U.S. was Walter. Therefore, for purposes of illustration of key differences in migration experiences it is useful to compare Rachel and Walter as contrast cases. Rachel was selected because of her distinct experience of being infected with HIV through involuntary sexual contact and her experiences as an asylum seeker in Germany. Rachel was from a small African village and Walter was from a major metropolitan city in the U.S. Despite the expected advantages that Walter may have had coming from a powerful country and a large cosmopolitan city, both Rachel and Walter were in a new country and encountered difficulties in adjusting to their new institutional and life situations. For Rachel this occurred in the realm of asylum seeker law and for Walter in the world of medicine. This suggests that problems in navigating new institutionalized social space and the stress associated with the need to go through these institutionalized channels are important aspects in migrant's life experiences in host countries. People with HIV can experience problems in not only coping with new medical systems, but also with navigating immigration laws in order to regain control over their autonomy and the ability to choose the nature of their stay in a new place. Rachel's narrative demonstrated how important immigration law can be in shaping spatial and temporal aspects of life. Due to asylum seeker law, Rachel lost control over her broader spatial location (having to stay in East Germany versus West Germany) and her more localized space (having to live in an environment characterized by a lack of privacy).

Cultural and economic conditions in the country of origin can also play an important role in life experiences. Participants who came from African countries did not report a distrust of medicine in Germany. Many participants coming from economically disadvantaged areas expressed a positive view of German medical care as they compared the quality of care to the limited treatment they had access to in their home countries. In contrast, Walter demonstrated a strong suspicion of medicine and government. This may reflect a cultural phenomenon in the U.S. of distrust among African Americans towards the community of medicine, which is rooted in the history of American politics and medicine. The distrust of medicine among African Americans has been documented (La Veist 2002). Unethical practices in medical research and the government such as the Tuskegee Syphilis experiment, where African Americans were not given treatment and used as a control group in order to study the natural progression of syphilis for forty years, is a well-known example of institutionalized racism and unethical treatment of blacks by the American government. Conspiracy theories of the government creating HIV/AIDS as a form of population control especially targeted towards the African American community have also been documented (Ross et al. 2006). In the American health care system, racial relations between patients and the medical system, which are rooted in a context of deep distrust due to racism, have been related to patients' satisfaction with care (LaVeist and Nuru-Jeter 2002).

3.10.1.1   Country of Origin and Role of Historical Racism in Views of Medicine: Conceptions of Truth and Deception

Interestingly, although coming from Africa to Germany, Rachel, Nancy, and David did not discuss experiences of racism in Germany. In contrast, Walter's experiences in America explicitly shaped his view of the world and he demonstrated a strong need for information as he explained:

> "There was once a thing said 'How do you keep a black man dumb?' 'Put it in books' know what I'm saying? This was, when I grew up this is what was said you know what I'm saying? You know 'How do you keep a black man dumb?' 'Keep it in books' 'Black men don't read' [Transcript 1; lines 1079-1086].

This desire for information and to think critically can be traced to Walter's understanding of racism and of slavery in American history. Walter felt that without awareness people were subject to exploitation and control. Walter's approach to truth and the media was relevant to the important issue of why Walter chose the metaphor of an experiment to accomplish the task of making

HIV unreal. Why was HIV not seen as a form of divine punishment? Why was HIV not a dream as initially described by Chris? Why was Walter in an elaborate experiment fueled by those in positions of power in order to further the realm of medicine and the will of the government? The historical context and life history of Walter provide some insight into his choice of metaphor.

Walter was a black man raised in a major city in America. He was aware of racism and discrimination and viewed himself as an educated man who sought information and strove to attain a deeper sense of awareness. He also viewed himself as aware of issues that most people in society were not aware of. He studied conspiracy theory, distrusted government, and valued self-education. Walter used his music as his personal form of generativity and as a gift to transmit messages to those who he felt lived blindly in a world where they were controlled by the powerful and where they followed others without questioning the arrangements of their lives. The world to Walter was not as it appeared. There was something beneath the surface of everyday life which remained to be discovered. Walter had a need to know the truth, he strived to find this truth, he did not know what this truth truly was but its pursuit was a major driving force in his life. He touched on a context of racism as he grew up in America. Walter was quick to say that things were now different but that in the past information was hidden from blacks to keep them ignorant and powerless. However, the past appeared to still be very present to Walter because he expressed a sense of paranoia and deep desire to educate himself and others. Walter's world view was tied to his view of HIV.

Walter's need for information, his distrust of those in power, and his awareness of racism were related to his approach to life and view of HIV as an experiment. Walter wanted answers to "where," "how," and "why" HIV was now a part of his life. He expressed a need to understand the etiology of HIV, the processes involved, and the meaning or purpose of HIV. Walter needed answers to these questions in order for him to accept that he had HIV. He repeatedly brought up the woman he had unprotected sex with for three years who was not infected with HIV in his narrative to deny the reality of HIV. Therefore, the intersectionality of HIV with racial/ethnic status was made clear in the case of Walter. Reality rooted in collective and personal history of racism in the U.S. interacted with Walter's conceptions of HIV and medical care.

However, a discussion of race was absent from other narratives. Why did African participants not discuss race? For example, Rachel lived in East Germany upon her arrival in Germany, an area characterized by racial tension. It is not clear why Walter explicitly discussed his blackness while Rachel did not. The interviewer was a white American woman and so one possibility is that the African women felt more comfortable discussing gender-related issues such as pregnancy and intimate relationships with a female interviewer than race. However, David came from an African country and did not discuss racism in his interview so a discussion of race did not appear to be dependent on gender. Walter may have brought up the issue of race because of my background as an American and he may have felt more comfortable discussing American politics and history as they related to racism to someone from his native country. Also, Walter came from a context where racism towards African Americans is an ongoing debate. Racism was more central in his awareness as he used his language and rhetoric purposefully to express himself. Unlike the other participants, Walter refused to view his HIV infection as a personal issue and instead used his argumentation to frame HIV as a politicized problem. Walter's orientation towards reality involved multiple social worlds. His distrust and suspicion manifested themselves in the realm of medicine, music, and entertainment. This illustrates how biographical position rooted in historical conditions (in this case the condition of racism) can be related to world view and orientation towards multiple facets of life. Indeed, stigma is rooted in history and rapid global economic changes, which have intensified inequality, emphasize the intersectionality between different forms of inequality such as race, immigration status, and HIV (Parker and Aggleton 2003).

3.10.1.2 Migration Experiences: Asylum Seeker Social Policy and Barriers to U.S. Travel

Prior research has found that people with HIV can experience discrimination in immigration (Parker et al. 2002). Rachel did not feel that there were laws that were especially targeted against people with HIV in Germany. Rather, she felt that the legal issues she encountered were unrelated to her HIV status. However, she allowed room for a subjective element in bureaucratic decision making but then moved away from this possibility. I probed further into the issue of legal difficulties and asked Rachel if dealing with the legal issues on top of everything else made things harder and she explained that her experiences as an asylum seeker had problematized her experiences. Although Rachel did not feel that people with HIV faced special legal issues in Germany, she did feel that the legal issues she had to navigate in as an asylum seeker did in fact make her life more difficult. Rachel's need to leave East Germany was illustrative of the potential ways in which immigration barriers can serve as a major stressor for people with HIV. Because institutional arrangements in asylum seeker law also shaped her access to economic resources, immigration contextualized her life experience with HIV.

This suggests that health is not divorced from the legislative institutional contexts which shape illness experience. Rather, as Rachel's story shows, asylum laws can have a profound impact on the life circumstances of migrants, shaping their living conditions, access to care, and importantly shaping the spatial and temporal aspects of their everyday lives. For example, Rachel was hundreds of miles away from her mother during her residence in East Germany. This spatial distance then shaped the temporal aspects of her life because she had to structure her time in order to be able to travel to meet her mother and then return to East Germany in time to register every month to receive her financial support.

Sources of support in navigating a new social space and culture can be essential in helping people to regain autonomy and to shape their lives in a manner that is spatially and temporally suited to their everyday needs. Without her mother, Rachel may have not been able to transverse German culture and this new institutionalized structuring of time and space to fit her needs. Asylum law in Germany, specifically dispersal policy, forced Rachel to reside in an asylum seeker house with limited privacy. Rachel described what it was like for her to take her medication during her stay at the asylum seeker house:

> "I couldn't stay there alone [...] there were many people and I used to hide my papers so nobody would see them under the bed [...] there was no privacy [...] medications ah were in the eh I used to have them in the bag so I was lucky these people they were like middle eastern they used to steal in this place in the house at that time (-) they didn't steal [...] I used to just go to toilet and I take my tablets." [Transcript 2, lines 481-498]

Rachel took special precautions to conceal her HIV status from her roommates and this was described as stressful to do in a context of limited privacy. She added that she was "lucky" because the Middle Eastern people in the house did not steal. Perhaps racial relations between immigrants are an important aspect of the migration experience. Therefore, additional analyses examining the experiences of people from other countries of origin and of a different racial background could help clarify how country of origin and race/ethnicity shape experiences living in Germany and migration experiences as they relate to living with HIV. In addition, taking medication emerged as an important daily routine. I asked Rachel if it made her feel uncomfortable to have to hide her medication and to take it in secret and Rachel responded that she felt more comfortable being able to take her medication in the privacy of her home. Similar to Rachel, Nancy came to Germany from an African country but did not report staying in an asylum seeker home. Nancy came to Germany in the late 1990s and was married in Germany and also worked with children. After Nancy discovered that she had HIV, she was concerned about immigration issues. Nancy had to get a visa for a permanent stay in Germany. Nancy explained that if someone works in Germany they could get a permanent stay but that she was not sure how to handle this issue because she had HIV and no one knew.

Travel emerged as a dimension of participants' life experiences. International travel and migration experiences were prevalent with even native Germans reporting international travel to the U.S. and other countries. For example Arthur, a man native to Germany, made cross-cultural comparisons and had traveled to numerous countries. Travel may facilitate the construction of cross-cultural comparisons and increase social awareness of cultural norms and institutions. Immigration law can however hinder people's ability to travel. Arthur discussed how he had to hide his HIV status in order to travel to the U.S. and how immigration law forced him to leave his apartment in a major city in the U.S. and to never return to the country:

> "Traveled to South America (-) traveled to North America (-) I lived in [major metropolitan area in the U.S.] for about eight years as a tourist more or less coming and going not as a resident because the American immigrant rights are a little funny for me and at the end I had a problem because an officer at the airport asked me why do I come so often to the U.S. and then I told him that I'm retired (-) I can look after myself financially and so on and I got lots of friends over there and he said "Ok" that was it (-) asking me silly things like what gang do I belong to? And why do I travel to North and South America as well? And I think he was probably guessing that I was a drug trafficking guy it was fine (-) then I quit my apartment I shared with friends over there and I came back home and I never came back to America." [Transcript 4, lines 52-61]

Arthur traveled to numerous countries and even lived as a resident in the U.S. for eight years. The place where Arthur lived was a large city with a substantial gay community, which is also known for having favorable weather, an emphasis on entertainment, and a more liberal political atmosphere. Importantly, Arthur discussed a major problem he encountered with the U.S. immigration system, which prevented him from living in the U.S. and forced him to return to Europe. He described an encounter with an officer at the airport who questioned him about his frequent traveling and how he responded to the officer by explaining that he was financially secure, retired, and had many friends in America. Arthur described the many questions the officer asked him. Was he a gang member? Why did he also travel to South America? Was he a drug trafficker? Arthur found these questions to be "silly" suggesting a sense of frustration. When I asked if he had ever had any legal trouble with immigration Arthur told:

"Probably (-) in my mind (-) for instance when I was going to America for three months I had to take my medication and if the custom people would have saw that in my luggage which occasionally happened (-) not going through all of it (-) but going through some of it and they might have had the possibility to trace back what kind of medication it was or just simply ask (-) if I would tell them (-) stay to the truth and I would have told them 'HIV' I would have had a problem (-) because of the form I-64 from the American immigration they ask me about being a Nazi (-) I'm born after the second World War so I can't be a Nazi from (-) from birth like (-) and they ask you silly questions about (pause) well they're not silly questions about being contagious for health (-) and HIV is a contagious thing and should they bring it up in the immigration office they say 'No you're not allowed to enter my territory' so you had to lie (-) It's different now because it's a universal thing that they have to (-) different governments have to allow HIV-positive traveling around the world (-) but at certain times it was different (-) you might have had problems coming out (-) open that you're HIV-positive." [Transcript 4, lines 306-319]

Arthur discussed the danger in bringing his HIV medication with him to stay in the U.S. for a period of three months and how if his medication were to be found he would have had trouble entering the country. He brought in dialogue as he explained that U.S. immigration asked him numerous questions. Arthur's German citizenship therefore was intrinsically tied to German history and was related to American views of Germany based on their understanding of history. The next issue was if Arthur had HIV, which Arthur had to lie about in order to enter the country. Arthur also discussed specific immigration forms demonstrating his experience with travel and immigration law. Consistent with the reality of U.S. immigration law, which was amended in 2010, Arthur felt that in the past HIV prevented people from entering the U.S. At the time of our interview he felt that numerous countries have to allow people with HIV to enter their territories and that the situation had changed. However, Arthur has never returned to the U.S. Furthermore, recent events in the U.S have been reported where people with HIV have been unable to enter the country, suggesting that discrimination against PLWHA in immigration remains an issue despite the policy change (Kremer 2012).

Traveling to the U.S. was common among the white European participants. The African participants reported more migration experiences to Germany and Walter, the only American participant interviewed in Germany, also reported traveling back and forth between the U.S. and Germany. Participant's experiences suggested that both nations' migration policies can be problematic for PLWHA. Dispersal programs targeted towards asylum seekers in Germany may have an unintended consequence of socially isolating HIV-positive migrants from their families at a critical time when they need support. Immigration law in the United States also presents a unique challenge for PLWHA because it can severely restrict travel and prevent integration into American society. Despite an increased awareness of how HIV can be transmitted, the U.S. has taken a conservative approach to immigration law as it applies to people with HIV. Migration experiences played important roles in contextualizing participants' experiences. Experienced stigma in the form of institutionalized immigration policy restricted participants' autonomy and ability to travel. Issues of restriction in travel, lack of freedom in living conditions, and more proximate conditions of a lack of privacy and fear of traveling with medication contextualized life experiences. Furthermore, Arthur's discussion of having to hide his medication when traveling and Rachel's descriptions of having to take her medication in secrecy while staying in the asylum seeker home were problematic. Medication use emerged as an important part of daily life. For example, both Rachel and Nancy discussed having to deal with the questions their children asked them about their medication use and health. Because medication taking emerged as an important facet of participants' daily lives, medication use and views of medical care are discussed next.

3.10.2   Views of Medical Care

Importantly, unlike Rachel, George, and David, Walter's health had not declined since his diagnosis. Accordingly, he did not view physicians as essential to his survival. Instead, Walter had a distrustful view of physicians as being part of the experiment where he felt he had been placed against his will. Therefore, health status may be an important dimension shaping how patients view medical treatment. Walter couldn't articulate why, but deep within in him was the undeniable feeling that he was being betrayed, and his betrayal was related to his conception of HIV as an experiment. As Walter discussed his view of the clinic, he remained in an active mode of thinking but blended this subtly with elements of passivity, suggesting feelings of betrayal and a loss of control.

Views of medicine can be shaped by not only health status and prior medical treatment experience, but also by the intersection of race/ethnicity and country of origin. The black participants who migrated from Africa even early in age to Europe did not report distrustful views of medicine. Was this difference due to African migrants' more existential need for quality medical treatment as compared to American patients who come from a developed nation? Perhaps need for treatment shaped patients' processes of meaning making and coping with racial tensions and relations, thus shaping their view of medicine. The socio-cultural context of racial relations and medical care may converge in shaping views of medicine. For example, Rachel's need for survival and treatment and her comparison of her medical care in Africa to her treatment in Germany suggests that Rachel felt that her medical care in Germany was an improvement on her past care and felt that the doctors here were supportive, knowledgeable, and a source of care and information. Unlike Walter, Rachel accepted her need for medical care and her role as a patient.

Rachel was faced with the need to survive and to overcome the possibility of death. Rachel viewed physicians as being necessary to her survival and her trust in medicine was driven by her desire to live. Despite living in a context of poverty, violence, and separation from her family Rachel still had the desire to carry on and to not give up on life. As a victim of sexual violence, Rachel could have chosen to disregard her health and lost her will to live and yet she still maintained her desire to live. Was this an instinctual desire? Or did Rachel still have hope at her young age that life could be different and that there was something left to keep fighting for? Rachel described her medical care in Africa as she explained how she was close to death at the time she sought medical care in her native country. Rachel's sickness came suddenly and her health worsened every day. Rachel faced a dilemma in treating her HIV and explained that she did not have access to effective medication. Problems with the access and quality of care were elaborated by Rachel entered a description of health care in her native country as she described her care by physicians as somewhat neglectful and uninvolved.

Rachel explicitly stated that the health care in her native African country was different than that of Germany. Rachel's description of the doctors in her village was negative she did not see the doctors as being very interested in their patients' health or reasons for pain. There was a lack of medicine and yet she had been instructed to take "tablets." This suggests that perhaps pain medications were the main source of treatment for an array of diseases and that the medical system was not sufficiently equipped to treat HIV effectively. Nancy also described the health care in her respective native African country in a similar manner as Rachel. Nancy felt that back at home someone could visit a physician but the physician was not a specialist. A physician could provide medication but the care was not as good as in Germany. Specialization of medicine was framed in a positive light. Perhaps, Rachel and Nancy's histories of care in their native countries shaped their expectations of their care in Germany. Both Rachel and Nancy had a positive view of medicine and the doctors at the clinic. Indeed,

Rachel's and Nancy's descriptions of their medical care in Germany were framed in a more positive manner. Rachel also described her time in a hospital in Eastern Germany when she became very ill and had to be hospitalized. The only people at this time that Rachel trusted were her mother and her physicians. Describing this part of her life was hard for Rachel as she was close to tears.

At that time, Rachel was in a position where she felt extremely dependent upon medical treatment for her survival. Rachel at the time of the interview was seeking care at the clinic and thus had experienced treatment from numerous physicians in different countries and even in different cities in Germany. David was very young upon his arrival to Germany from his native African country and did not report any experiences in the African health care system. However, David had a very positive view of his current medical care and he reported satisfaction with his physicians and medical insurance and made a favorable comparison of the German health care system to other health care systems in the U.S. and in third world countries.

3.10.2.1   Medical Treatment as a Reminder of HIV

Walter and Nancy discussed how seeking treatment and taking medication served as reminders of their HIV status. For example, Walter explained:

> "It becomes a burden at times (-) I mean I don't think about it every day or all the time (-) but I do think a lot (-) like I wake up every morning (-) I get up and take this fucking pill (-) you know? I gotta take this pill every morning and when my pill runs out I got to make sure I call these people and they give me another dose of these pills (-) **just in case**." [Transcript 1, lines 525-529]

Walter's HIV treatment was a daily reminder of his HIV status. Every day began with taking "this fucking pill." This expression indicates his dislike and frustration of the need to take medication daily. In the unfolding of Walter's future life with HIV, medication use may be an important issue that needs special attention. Walter did not trust his medication and viewed it as potentially toxic and injecting him with foreign and ambiguous material. Medication was a reminder of Walter's new life with HIV, which carried the burden of secrecy. Walter emphasized "just in case" suggesting that he had doubts regarding an actual need for adhering to his medication. Just in case, Walter took "this fucking pill." There was an element of aggression and resistance because Walter seemed to resent his medication.

Nancy explained that at the moment of the interview she was feeling "down" and how in the past thinking about her HIV. Nancy described that every time she had to go to the clinic to see the doctor or have blood drawn she was very depressed. Nancy was so distraught in the beginning of her new life with HIV that her first physician sent her to a psychologist for help. Rachel also reported feeling uncomfortable and fearful of seeking care when she first was diagnosed. This suggests that for newly diagnosed patients seeking care and taking medication can serve as reminders of HIV and can be depressing and stressful.

In contrast, although Chris had only been living with HIV for one year he told that he not have any regrets because he felt that nothing changed. He was healthy and not on medication. His diagnosis allowed him to experience "real love" and to find "emotions" and "support" that he had always searched for before and never experienced. The moment of crisis allowed Chris to experience true love because his partner accepted him and stood by him in his time of need and did not change the way he treated him. Chris explained how not having to take medication was involved in his daily awareness of HIV:

> "This disease right now isn't really like affecting my life negative (-) um like so my family knows (-) my some of my close friends know and um that's about it (-) it's like I really forget it (-) that I have it(-) cause it's not affecting me (-) like I'm not on medication or anything so it's (--) in the back of my head like I know it's there but like it's like far (-) far (-) far back so so not aware everyday." [Transcript 3, lines 48-55]

Chris did not feel that HIV had a major negative impact on his life and he disclosed his HIV status to his family and close friends. While medication use was not an issue for Chris, the desire to "have a normal life" and to have children was presented as an important issue but was then minimized. Chris minimized problems in his narrative as opposed to Walter who problematized his troubles and discontent. While Chris may seem to be more accepting of HIV than Walter, his minimization of problems may actually represent a form of denial. Chris appeared to still be wrestling with his new life with HIV but was acting to portray his self as healthy and "normal." Walter completely buried his awareness. Interestingly, he buried this awareness despite his feelings that awareness was important and that it was important to not be ignorant and to look deeper into the meaning of reality. This suppressed awareness was on the edge of his reality and so his method of suppression (the experiment construction) may have been on the verge of collapse. Chris' awareness was far back in the recesses of his mind and he did not feel that HIV was in his daily awareness context. Both Walter and Chris were healthy, living with HIV for one year, and similar in terms of age and gender. Chris seemed to have more acceptance but did not think of his disease everyday. Walter had to take "this fucking pill" everyday, which was a reminder of HIV that he constructed into the belief that his medication was a scientific mode of keeping a virus within him. This construction helped Walter to cope with this forced reminder of a disease which he denied existed.

Therefore, daily routines and activities linked to HIV can serve as reminders of HIV. The routine nature of medication taking was described by David who had system for taking his medication that was based in numbers. David used a "10, 10, 10, 10 in morning 10 in evening" system for organizing his daily medication regimen (Sequential Report 8, p. 5). David reflected on how initially he wanted to take his pills at the exact time because he was a perfectionist. David used his phone to set an alarm and always brought his pills with him. Importantly, David explained that this routine was a process of learning. Initially, David took many pills, which he hated to do and still recalled the colors of the pills (blue, white, and orange) and his hatred for them. A major issue for David involved in having to take so many pills was his fear that others would see him taking his medication. This was a heavy thing to deal with, David hated the color, he hated the time, he told his physician and they changed his medication. The reduction in the amount of pills in his treatment regimen to three in the morning and to two in the evening was a major improvement for David. The color had changed, now his medication was only two colors. David felt that taking multiple medications was a problem because he would have to try to explain why he was taking them. Taking medication was described as a symbolic marker of HIV status and illness that forced HIV into daily awareness and had the potential to expose the secret status of HIV.

Medication use can be problematic for patients because not only is it a daily reminder of HIV, but the fear of being seen taking HIV medication and having to explain their pill-taking was described as being uncomfortable and anxiety inducing. Similar to David, Rachel discussed feelings of discomfort taking her medication in a context of limited privacy while staying at an asylum seeker home and her relief at being able to take her medication in a more private setting in her own home. The dimensions of medication use as a reminder of HIV and inducing a fear of being seen taking medication emerged as important aspects of daily life, which should be further examined in research focusing on the issue of medication adherence.

3.10.2.2   Concerns in Medical Care

Language barriers were negotiated in medical care. Rachel discussed her experiences seeking care before she was able to speak German as difficult. Rachel explained that language was an important factor in her preference for certain physicians and that she learned German in order to be more autonomous when seeking care for her HIV. Before Rachel learned German she used a creative approach to communicate with her physicians. By using the commonly understood symbol of "HIV" Rachel was able to communicate with the doctors at some level. The understanding of "HIV" across cultures shows the global influence and awareness of HIV. Rachel felt a need to be more independent so that she would not need to always have to depend upon someone else to translate for her. This highlights the importance of communication between patients and physicians in interaction. Rachel viewed mastering the German language as a means to more effective and efficient care seeking. Similarly, Nancy discussed the importance of language. Nancy wanted to talk to people who were from her native country about language and translate things for them because she felt that many people from her country could speak only their native languages or English and they were afraid to take their medication because they did not know who to talk to.

3.10.2.3   Making Comparisons between the U.S. and Germany

When making sense of the world of HIV, comparisons were made between the U.S. and Germany. Such comparisons may have been made partly because of my role as an American researcher. However, the issue of cross-cultural comparisons was made without prompting. Participants utilized comparisons throughout their narratives as they reconstructed their biographies. Comparisons to past and present were made including: past social context to present social context, past personal context to present situation, and past to present self. Participants often compared: their lives before their diagnosis to their lives after diagnosis, their views of people with HIV to their views of themselves, and their views of HIV to different illnesses. The use of national comparisons suggests that participants also considered broader societal arrangements as they made sense of HIV.

For example, Arthur preferred living in Europe and the European system to the American system. Importantly, when he is discussed a "system" he was referring to multiple types of systems, the system regulating retirement benefits and social security and the system regulating health care coverage (Transcript 4, line 133). This suggests that Arthur recognized these different systems as having interplay with one another and that these policies had an impact on his financial and medical well-being. Arthur also emphasized the importance of economic resources for medical care and the medical-industrial complex:

> "The medication I'm getting costs about (-) I don't know (-) $2,000 a month and if you have to have your own healthcare you pay full or have to pay your medication yourself (-) who can afford that? Like people in Africa for instance what they have to pay (-) it's a completely different thing they can't afford it (-) unless the companies like Pfizer and Paxel or whatever make generic or allow (--) the companies to use it at a much less rate." [Transcript 4, lines 143-149]

Arthur recognized the major issue of the discrepancy between the price of medication and people's actual resources to obtain their medication. Arthur framed this in the context of the U.S. system of Health Maintenance Organizations (HMOs) and pharmaceutical industries that have a strong vested interest in not allowing for the availability for cheaper, generic versions of medication, which makes it very difficult for people to be able to afford treatment. David also made comparisons between Germany and the U.S. in terms of their healthcare systems. Specifically, David emphasized how the German health care system allowed PLWHA to be able to afford their medication and to maintain a better quality of life as compared to other nations. David explained how the U.S. is one of the richest countries in the world but has, in his view, the worst health care. He did not understand how people with HIV lived in the U.S. David was very proud to be German, to live in Germany, and to not have to worry about his health insurance. David felt that he had a very good job and income and did not have to pay for his medication and felt that not having to pay for his medication was a "big freedom" (Sequential Report 8, p. 4). David without being prompted emphasized:

> "Can you imagine having a problem with the medication? Having problem with money? With the insurance, whatever to cover the medication? Then having the same problems at home with families, problems with your culture, religion, problems being ahm HIV-positive, problems being homosexual, being all these things? **That would kill you** all that. All those things are too much. But the medication system, the health care system here that's one thing I don't need to take care about." [Sequential Report 8, p. 4]

Therefore, the German health care system was a major help to David who felt that living with HIV involved many difficult aspects of life. He could not imagine living with HIV without the financial freedom and support the German health care system provided. David elaborated on the issue of the cost of medication for HIV when asked how he felt he would be doing if Germany did not have this health care system. David responded that he was thinking about that same issue. With his income he could afford the medication. The pills he took just one type of medication cost 600 euros, the others cost about 800 euros. The cost of his medication would be about 1200-1500 euros a month just for the pills without seeing the doctor. Because David had a high income he could afford to buy the medication himself but then he would have to go back to a one room apartment, he would have to sell his car, he would have to cut a lot of things out of his life, which made his life easier. David would have to cut a lot of things just to cover the bill for pills hoping nothing else would happen because he wouldn't be able to afford it. For example, he explained when he had to have a tumor removed from his back he wouldn't be able to pay that bill of 100,000 euros. David said this was the exact problem in the U.S., he argued that people have to sell their homes to get health care. David explained that for other people that he knew from Helping Hand they would not be able to live without the financial support their health care provided in Germany. David felt that these people would die without their health insurance because they would not be able to afford the medication or health care.

Arthur was aware of global issues as he discussed Africa and the difficulties people in Africa can have in being able to obtain treatment due to the high cost of HIV medication, widespread poverty, and social inequality. David also felt that most people with HIV in third world countries probably die but hoped that in the U.S. people don't die. Arthur identified a solution to this issue, which was for the pharmaceutical companies to allow for cheaper generic versions of HIV medication or to lower the cost of medication. However, this solution was highly political and the companies involved have an enormous amount of power and a strong vested interest to prevent such a solution from occurring. A solution to the high cost of medical treatment of HIV may therefore require a collaborative effort between pharmaceutical companies, governmental agencies, insurance companies, and physicians.

3.10.2.4   Comorbidity of HIV, Physical and Mental Illness

Another important concern discussed by participants was the comorbidity of health problems for aging patients with HIV. Cancer, strokes, memory problems, and cardiovascular issues were reported by participants. These concerns have major implications for the health care of the first cohort of an aging population with HIV. Sarah described a recent stroke:

"I had this operation and then six months later I had the stroke (-) which **may** be connected with HIV they can't say but they're not very sure although they can't say it's HIV itself or the treatment because I don't have any other risk factors I don't have overweight (-) I don't have a disfamiliar disposition (-) I don't have very high blood pressure so what else? I don't smoke and I don't I don't drink (-) and so the only thing which was left was the HIV (-) although they can't say if it's HIV itself or if it's the treatment." [Transcript 5, lines 541-546]

After Sarah had an operation for her uterus cancer she had a stroke that the doctors believed was potentially due to either her HIV or her HIV medication because she had no other risk factors for stroke. This prompted me to ask more about her medical treatment for HIV and to ask if she has had any problems with her medication or any side effects. Sarah felt she had no bad side effects due to her HIV medication and yet she recently suffered from a stroke that her physicians attributed to either her HIV or her medication. I asked more about her health and treatment. Sarah responded that her HIV therapy had not been problematic for the past ten to fifteen years and that the only alterations to her medication regimen had to do with her cholesterol levels. Cholesterol problems were the only issue she reported having with her medication despite the possibility that her treatment could have contributed to her stroke. Because Sarah discussed various health issues I probed more about her health problems. Sarah attributed her health problems to aging and related to her friends who did not have HIV and who were getting older and experiencing similar health problems. She also discussed how her health changed after menopause. Therefore, age-related health issues allowed Sarah to be able to relate her health to other people who did not have HIV, which may have helped to normalize the problems she experienced. Indeed, Sarah downplayed any connection HIV or her medication could have to her new health problems. Having cancer, a stroke, or high blood pressure can mean something very different for someone who does not have HIV. Sarah even told that her own experiences with HIV shaped her experiences dealing with her more recent health problems and framed her health problems in a positive way. These were problems that she did not have to hide and which she could relate to other people who were HIV-negative, which may have normalized these experiences and even given her a sense of comfort and relief as suggested by her description of cancer as a "relaxation." Sarah's description of cancer as a relaxation was very telling and revealed the heavy burden that the secret of HIV placed on Sarah's life. Sarah's experience of menopause also emphasizes the intersection of age, gender, and HIV in her treatment. Arthur also had lung cancer:

"It's a big thing but actually to me but looking backwards it was not so important like it looked at the time when I caught it because at that time I was fearing I would die [...] I have other problems like the heart (-) has nothing to do with the infection (-) I have a heart problems (-) I've got lung cancer now these are things which concern me more than HIV" [Transcript 4;lines 85-92].

Because Arthur lived with HIV for a long period of time the manner in which he separated the past from the present was notable. From his present state of mind, HIV was not especially salient to him, but he recalled his prior conceptions and how HIV used to be a major issue in his life when he was diagnosed and scared that he was going to die. Arthur's coping had a temporal aspect, as new information and experiences were sedimented in his life, the manner in which he framed his HIV changed. He took the perspectives of his current self and his past self when talking about how HIV was a part of his life. As he went through his narrative, he continuously related his current self to his past self as he situated himself to describe his long-term experiences with HIV. Arthur emphasized his age at diagnosis. He was in his forties when he was diagnosed with HIV and at the time of the interview he was in his early sixties. Arthur appeared to emphasize his age in order to emphasize that he had other health problems. He now had heart problems and lung cancer to manage. Older age even in the absence of HIV introduces a new host of health issues that need to be monitored. Heart health, cholesterol, arthritis, memory loss, and other chronic conditions began to develop among older participants.

Arthur was more concerned with his chronic heart problems and lung cancer than with his HIV. This suggests a temporal aspect to coping with illness because after years of living with HIV, Arthur had new health problems to deal with and thus HIV was minimized in his discussion of his health. Arthur did not complain of pain or discuss his moment of diagnosis of his heart problems or cancer even though these were more recent. This may be either due to a social desirability bias because he was aware that the topic of this study was HIV or it is possible that HIV presented more of an existential crisis where he had to face the possibility of death than his more recent diagnoses. Perhaps his earlier coping with HIV even made him more resilient to his new diagnoses because he has faced the possibility of death before and managed to live a long life in spite of his HIV. Arthur's resilience to HIV may have been a source of strength in the face of cancer because he faced death before and had the life experience of managing a chronic illness that initially was conceived of as a death sentence. Similarly, Sarah explained how she was not as shocked by her more recent health problems. In contrast to HIV, Sarah did not report feeling shocked or having an extreme reaction to her cancer and the necessary operation she had to undergo for treatment and she explicitly stated that this was because she "was used to having a deadly illness, or severe illness, threatening one." Therefore, living long-term with HIV can actually build resiliency in the face of a threatening illness. Importantly, Sarah also sought treatment for mental health problems and discussed public conceptions of HIV and mental illness in terms of cross-cultural comparisons based on her experiences traveling and her understanding of German history:

> "I mean don't forget that was twenty years ago (-) it was also something else at that time probably having a therapy (-) there's a big difference between Germany and USA also (-) this is something um which also is uh can lead to a stigma (-) at least people think that (-) this is partly also due to Germany's own history (-) euthanasia and everything in the Third Reich (-) they say so at least (-) it seems to be a reasonable thought (-) and still today (-) going to a 'shrink' (laughs) (-) going to psychotherapy is not very normal here." [Transcript 5, lines 257-264]

Sarah explained that she had made a conscious decision to do therapy and brought in the social context of the time when she first initiated her search for a therapist twenty years ago. A difference between the present and the past and how attitudes towards the controversial issue of mental illness have changed was emphasized. Sarah also made an international and cultural distinction between Germany and the U.S. She felt that in Germany attitudes towards getting treatment for mental health issues were more stigmatizing than in the U.S. Sarah supported her argument that Germany was less accepting of mental illness by linking German public conceptions of mental illness to Germany's history. Sarah's own personal experience in seeking therapy was rooted in the cultural context of Germany's unique history and she herself acknowledged the link between her personal experiences and history as she made a distinction between German and American attitudes. Sarah felt that people feared those with mental illness and those seeking treatment for mental health problems. Although she felt that in the past attitudes towards mental illness were more negative than in the present, she still felt that these negative attitudes towards mental illness were an issue. Sarah explained how seeking therapy was considered deviant and not "normal." Sarah had an interest in psychotherapy and read numerous pieces on the subject indicating that she had an active interest in seeking information about psychotherapy and an interest in self-exploration. Her psychotherapy was pivotal to her life as she explained "I think it was the best thing I could have done." Sarah had a very positive view of psychotherapy and felt that it is a major factor in her own personal resilience and success. I asked about the difference between German and American attitudes towards therapy and she explained:

"I have some American friends and all these things and I've been to America a few times and I know that in the states it is quite uh (-) seen as something as much more normal belonging to daily life (-) and at least in bigger cities (-) talk about (-) not in say the rural parts of Wisconsin or something (laughs) of course not (-) there are differences also (-) but eh (-) as I (-) as I noticed myself (-) or as I heard in conversations and all these things (-) this is handled much more lightly (-) much more uh you know (-) without any prejudices (-) and Germany people are still scared."
[Transcript 5, lines 275-280]

Sarah traveled to America and had American friends and based on her experiences observing others' conversations, American culture, and what she heard from her American friends, she felt that in the U.S. seeking help for mental health issues was more socially acceptable. Both Sarah and Arthur discussed their travels and made international comparisons between Germany and the U.S. This highlights the role of travel as a means of facilitating an awareness of cultural differences and reflections on how cultural differences can have implications for the understanding of one's native country and institutionalized systems. For example, Arthur discussed made cross-cultural comparisons as he described health, finance, and immigration policies and a new understanding of public attitudes towards deviant behavior, such as the decriminalization of his gay sexuality. Similar to Sarah, Arthur reflected on public attitudes towards mental health treatment and the historical roots of public attitudes in German culture.

However, in the U.S. mental illness remains a stigmatized status with national surveys of public attitudes of mental illness showing that the American public demonstrates a fear of people with mental illness, a desire for social distance, perceptions of dangerousness, and even a desire to socially control people with mental health issues (Mossakowski et al. 2011). Then why did Sarah feel that Germany was even more apprehensive regarding the issue of mental illness? Did she experience any negative reactions by others who may know about her psychotherapy? Or was she more aware of the cultural differences between the U.S. and Germany because was an educated woman who traveled between the two nations where she observed these differences in public opinion in the daily life of her American friends? Sarah's discussion of mental illness stigma raised another issue of the comorbidity of mental health issues with HIV.

Being diagnosed with HIV was a major shock to the majority of the participants interviewed, which suggests that when being confronted with HIV, people may benefit from receiving therapy and support from therapists, psychologists, or psychiatrists. However, if mental illness is another socially deviant status, the fear of being seen utilizing such services or the internalization of a negative attitude towards therapy could be biographically disruptive and inhibit positive well-being. This also highlights the constellation of stressors involved in HIV. Sarah was not only someone with HIV, she was a widow of a man who she believed had been unfaithful, a mother of two children, a working professional, and was a patient of psychotherapy. What did the constellation of all of these social statuses with their own benefits and stressors mean for Sarah's health and well-being? The constellation of multiple stressors rooted in the structural arrangement inherent in her social roles as they were present in Sarah's life was consistent with Pearlin's (1989) conception of stress proliferation. Pearlin's (1989) fundamental proposition was that stress cannot be studied in isolation and that multiple stressors can have an overlap and interplay affecting coping and well-being. Therefore, as the case of Sarah illustrates, qualitative analysis can be especially useful for examining the utility of sociological paradigms of the stress process.

While mental illness is a distinct phenomenon from HIV, studies on the stigma of mental illness indicate some factors related to stigma are relevant to the current analysis. Perceptions of dangerousness, assessed by likelihood of violence or harm to others or to the person afflicted with mental illness, have been found to play instrumental roles in increasing preferences for social distance and for support of coercive treatment, such as forced medication use and hospitalization of people with mental illness (Corrigan et al. 2003; Mossakowski et al. 2011). Fear of infection from HIV can be conceptualized as a parallel perception of dangerousness of PLWHA. Both mental illness and HIV share similar characteristics, they are deviant conditions and their causes can be considered by others to be due to a defect or fault in the person afflicted. Indeed, attributing the cause of mental illness to biological causes, such as a genetic problem or a chemical balance in the brain was not found to be sufficient in reducing negative attitudes towards mental illness (Mossakowski et al. 2011). Similarly, the widespread anti-stigma efforts geared towards HIV may not be fully effective in reducing HIV stigma by providing people only with medical information about routes of transmission via unprotected sex and intravenous drug use. Instead, previous research and the current analysis suggest that in order to reduce HIV stigma, perceptions of dangerousness, as indicated by fear of infection, must be reduced in combination with decreasing attributions of blame that can serve to shame those with HIV and stigmatize them. People can come across HIV in a number of ways that are beyond their immediate control. Trusting a sexual partner and forced sexual contact are modes of transmission that are not widespread in public discussions of HIV.

Also, because HIV can be a catalyst for an existential crisis as indicated by participants' shock and distress at their diagnoses, the issues of mental health and

HIV can be closely intertwined. Engagement in social support and educational programs such as Helping Hand played a pivotal role in participants' coping with HIV. Seeking mental health treatment was also a major factor in Sarah's empowerment and ability to cope positively with her HIV, but Sarah felt that in Germany seeking mental health treatment was socially deviant:

> "People (-) as I said (-) don't know what psychotherapy is (-) not very uh well it's not the normal thing (-) it's just always with some um maybe prejudices (-) you could (-) you could say that as people are more or less scared of it (-) it's not just someone says 'Ah I have the feeling I have to go see somebody and handle my problems or whatever' this is not uh daily routine here." [Transcript 5, lines 284-287]

Psychotherapy was considered as something that was not normal and which people held a prejudice against due to their fear and lack of information. Sarah explained her view that seeking therapy was not normative in German society and that people did not recognize their mental health problems and take action to seek care or discuss their care because this was not part of the normative daily routine. Therefore, Sarah was engaged in an activity for years that she felt was not accepted by the status quo. Yet psychotherapy was something that she felt very positively about and that she felt had truly helped her to find her inner strength. Did Sarah experience any conflicts with her conception of therapy and public conceptions that she felt were fearful and prejudiced? Sarah did not explicitly discuss this issue but because she took the effort to observe other cultures and to understand public attitudes this suggests that this was a salient issue for her. Despite the negative attitudes which she felt German society had towards therapy, she continued to seek care for years, which indicated a strong interest and commitment to her mental health. Sarah elaborated on public conceptions of mental illness and their formation in German history:

> "That might really have to do something with a special history cause in the time of the Third Reich they had [...] the so-called (-) they find lives not worth living (-) these were people having handicaps (-) people especially with mental handicaps and these people were also brought to the concentration camps (-) so having someone in the family like that (-) having someone like that in the family (-) could be a very well difficult thing to cope with either you have to keep them back or it could happen that they really came and got them (-) and this a bad chapter of German history but it belongs to that and so some people think it might really have something to do with these things in history that today people think psychotherapy as something with mental health (-) mental health (-) mental health it's something very sensible (--) something very sensitive subject it might have maybe some connection." [Transcript 5, lines 296-310]

Sarah emphasized how in the U.S. she felt that seeking mental health services was a part of daily life and was more routine and thus normalized. In contrast, in Germany she felt that the mass murder of people with "mental handicaps" during World War II had a lasting impact on public attitudes towards mental illness. During World War II, people had to conceal family members with mental illness or else they would be brought into concentration camps and killed. Sarah felt that Germany had a "special history" and that World War II was "a bad chapter of German history." Therefore, Sarah described how public conceptions of mental illness appeared to be rooted in historical events. The connection she made between Germany's special history and public attitudes towards mental health and how this related to her own personal history of seeking mental health counseling indicates that Sarah was very much attuned to the historical and cultural relevance of her own life circumstances. The intersection of the experiences of HIV, stress, and mental health was grounded in the cultural and historical context of Sarah's life. Life experiences of living with HIV were deeply embedded in personal history and were grounded in the historical and social context of participants' lives. Engaging in a comparative analysis helped to generate important insights into participants' personal histories and their socio-historical context.

4 Discussion

4.1 Summary of Findings

The major aim of this research project was to examine how PLWHA experience their illness and in which ways HIV becomes a part of one's biography. I examined under what conditions trajectories of suffering could be overcome and what types of biographical action schemes were related to coping with HIV. PLWHA in both Frankfurt and Miami emphasized the importance of the social context of their diagnosis and the mode of HIV transmission as contextual conditions, which framed their HIV experiences. HIV became a meaningful part of participants' biographies, fundamentally altering their conceptions of HIV, mortality, self, truth, and the spiritual. The acceptance of a new life with HIV was contextualized by biographical experience. For those who could clearly identify the cause of their HIV infection, whose social positions were most consistent with prevailing conceptions of HIV, and who felt responsible for HIV transmission appeared to more readily come to terms with their HIV infection. HIV specialist care, medical insurance coverage for treatment, and access to HIV medication were highly valued by participants and were important aspects of their HIV treatment, facilitating coping with HIV and improving quality of life.

4.1.1 Biography and HIV as a Trajectory of Suffering

Consistent with my expectations, participants described HIV as both an initial threat to mortality upon diagnosis. They also had to contend with the shifting meaning of HIV as a chronic illness, which they had to come to terms with over time. Existing frames of reference were often challenged and deeply rooted challenges to existing schemes of meaning contributed to interviewee's struggles with meaning making to deal with the existential threat of HIV. This struggle was related to the negative symbolism surrounding HIV, which threatened people's conceptions of who they were and what they could become at a deep, existential level. Processes of meaning making were grounded in interviewees' local context, personal history, and broader societal conditions. Also, similar to the findings of previous studies, I found that HIV diagnosis was often stressful, shocking, and characterized by feelings of being thrown into a new life against one's will (Kelly et al. 1998; Safren et al. 2003). However, in some cases HIV diagnosis was described as almost expected due to histories of high risk behavior. Yet even when described as anticipated, elements of shock and stress were still present in participants' narratives.

HIV was experienced as a trajectory of suffering, which presented powerful existential threat to mortality, identity, and meaning (Riemann and Schütze 1991). Consistent previous biographical research, I found that participants, while overwhelmed by the suffering of HIV, were active in engaging in biographical work aimed at reconstructing their identities in response to their HIV status (Carricaburu and Pierret 1995). HIV was experienced as a trajectory of suffering that required participants to restructure their everyday lives, conceptions of themselves and of HIV, and to navigate their social worlds which had become framed in a context of danger in social interaction. My analysis emphasized the importance of symbolic meanings linked to HIV status and the role of the presentation of self in the negotiation of HIV disclosure. The social construction of social interaction and its relationship to the negotiation of social order and of the self are an enduring focus of sociological theory and research (Mead 1934; Strauss 1993; Blumer 1969; Giddens 1995; Goffman 1959). Danger and disruption emerged as essential characteristics of trajectories of suffering, which facilitated a bracketing of social reality and an analysis of the taken for granted patterns of social reality by both the researcher and interviewees in this study (Husserl and Brough 1991; Husserl 1964). The dramaturgical character of social interaction was heightened for participants in both samples who, in their desires to maintain a sense of normalcy and sameness in their social relationships, carefully negotiated their HIV disclosure. Bury (1982) made a similar analysis of chronic illness as biographical disruption as he argued that chronic illness was an experience that involves a disruption of existing forms of knowledge and daily life. Bury (1982) argued that chronic illness involved an awareness of worlds of pain and suffering and potential death, which for others without illness are merely distant possibilities. Furthermore, he contended that chronic illness forces individuals, their families, and social contacts to come face-to-face with the nature of their relationships and disrupts normal rules of reciprocity and social support (Bury 1982, p. 169).

My findings correspond to the characteristics of biographical disruption as proposed by Bury (1982) which include: (1) "the disruption of taken for-granted assumptions and behaviors; the breaching of commonsense boundaries" (2) "profound disruptions in explanatory systems normally used by people, such that a fundamental re-thinking of the person's biography and self-concept" (3) "the response to disruption involving the mobilization of resources, in facing an altered situation" (p. 169 f.). Others using a biographical approach to studying HIV have found that biographical reinforcement of identity can be a fundamental aspect of coming to terms with HIV (Carricaburu and Pierret, 1995). Carricaburu and Pierret (1995) found that PLWHA constructed meaning in their present lives by relating the present to their reconstructed individual life stories and collective pasts, which helped them to construct a new identity and to create a sense of continuity in their biographies. Similar to my results, the past was reconstructed in different ways depending on the mode of HIV transmission. This process of biographical reinforcement was "a reinforcement of their identities on the basis of what they had been before infection" (Carricaburu and Pierret 1995, p. 80).

4.1.2   Awareness of Discredibility and Epistemological Struggle

Although the concepts of stigma and social support inspired the initial research project, using the biographical approach generated unanticipated insights that fundamentally altered the initial research questions. Discussions regarding the nature of reality and truth emerged in both samples as interviewees discussed their conceptions of truth. Epistemological struggles with the nature of truth, knowledge, and reality emerged in both samples. Participants made distinctions between surface or superficial reality and the real, deeper reality, which was seen as being under the surface of external reality. This debate of the nature of truth suggests that participants struggled as HIV entered their biography and required them to shift their preexisting notions of reality. The distinction between surface and real reality in social interaction was emphasized in relation to interviewees' awareness that if they disclosed their HIV status their social relationships and interactions with others would be fundamentally altered. For example, some participants discussed overhearing people talking about HIV and staying silent as they expressed the feeling that others without HIV were ignorant about HIV and would not be able to understand their HIV condition. Participants' awareness of the potential for stigma emphasized HIV stigma as a discreditable stigma that could be concealed from others in social interaction (Goffman 1963). The awareness of the potential for stigma often was related to the decision to keep HIV a secret from others. The discreditable nature of HIV stigma emphasized the elements of danger in social interaction which were discussed by Anselm Strauss as he discussed Goffman and the process of status-forcing (1959):

"But you can be, and continually are, the unwitting agent of such status-forcing. Goffman, in writing of the constant danger of losing and causing loss of face, makes the point that during conversation everybody is 'in jeopardy'; because of the rules covering conversation, one is in constant danger of causing or receiving the 'affront.' The wider point at issue is that much more than affront and insult seem to be involved. Interaction carries the potential of unwitting as well as witting imputation of countless motives and character-to others and to self. It can be said consequently that the very nature of interaction implies the forcing of status. it is worth remembering that interaction not only puts everyone concerned in danger-actors and audience alike-but equally exposes everybody to transforming experiences that are more positive and creative in implication." (p. 84)

Accordingly, participants described an awareness of the potential for discredibility in their interactions with others and employed strategies to avoid status-forcing often by maintaining secrecy. HIV disclosure emerged as a fundamental aspect of living with HIV. Participants in both samples made distinctions between HIV-positive and HIV-negative communities as external referents. Disclosure was described as a difficult decision which involved a careful consideration of potential social losses, rejection, and delegitimization. This is consistent with prior qualitative research, which finds that PLWHA selectively disclose and often choose to keep their HIV a secret (Carricaburu and Pierret 1995; Pierret 2001). The division between the HIV-positive and -negative worlds was more pronounced in the Frankfurt sample. While participants in both samples often selectively disclosed to a few close relations, there were no reports of disclosing in the workplace among the Frankfurt sample. This difference could be due to sampling bias. Alternatively, while it is not possible to generalize, this difference may be due to people's professions and the local cultural context. Those who disclosed their HIV status publicly and in the workplace tended to either run their own businesses or were living in extremely disadvantaged socioeconomic positions.

Those who ran their own businesses may have had more autonomy and freedom in their careers, which could have encouraged them to take the risk of being open about their HIV status. Also, for those living in extreme poverty, they may have felt that they had less to lose by openly challenging negative stereotypes of HIV in their communities. Being open about HIV was an important phenomenon because not only did it help people in their personal life circumstances to feel empowered, but because it allowed for them to challenge the existing discourse surrounding HIV. Disclosure allowed HIV to enter the working world and to alter personal experience and gave it the potential to alter existing conceptions of HIV in public discourse. Alfred Schütz (Schütz 1962) described the working world as:

"Paramount over against the many other sub-universes of reality. It is the world of physical things including my body; it is the realm of my locomotions and bodily operations[...]permits me to carry through my plans, and enables me to succeed or to fail in my attempt to attain my purposes. By my working acts I gear into the outer world, I change it [...]the world of the working is the reality within which communication and the interplay of mutual motivation becomes effective." (p. 227)

Therefore, the decision to disclose, while dangerous, also had the potential to create positive change by altering social reality. Fear of stigma was a major barrier to disclosing HIV and thus had the potential to perpetuate marginalization. My findings suggest that a powerful resource for PLWHA was access to a collective identity in a supportive context. This could empower PLWHA to work to challenge their marginalized identities into activist identities or "project identities," which could change public discourse about HIV (Castells 1997; Parker and Aggleton 2003). Participation in support groups and involvement in meaningful relations of care provided social resources, which helped participants to construct a more positive view of their HIV status and to reduce their fear of stigma.

However, being open or going public with HIV had negative consequences, such as the loss of professional standing and career, rejection, and problems in finding and maintaining romantic relationships. Furthermore, because of the stress of being open about HIV, along with the experience of other numerous stressors, in some cases participants in this study decided to withdraw and to no longer be open about their HIV status. The decision to withdraw and to no longer fight to challenge negative stereotypes of HIV is problematic because it hinders the possibility for social change and empowerment. Future research is encouraged to further examine how the constellation of life experiences and conditions is related to the decision to go public with HIV and to remain open.

Furthermore, future efforts to combat the AIDS epidemic can be informed by the historical AIDS activism during the 1980s in the establishment of the Foundation for AIDS Research (AmfAR) in the U.S. AmfAR, an international, nonprofit organization, was created in a collaboration that merged two social worlds: the entertainment industry and science. The collaborations between actress Elizabeth Taylor and researcher Mathilde Krim gave a face to HIV/AIDS in public discourse and their efforts shaped political and social change and impacted social policy. For example, the Ryan White Act, which Elizabeth Taylor actively lobbied for was passed. The Ryan White Foundation remains the largest source of funding for HIV/AIDS treatment in the U.S. In fact, participants in Miami felt that the Ryan White program helped them to obtain treatment and to be able to maintain their medical care.

With the ongoing budgetary concerns regarding the funding of governmental programs, my results indicate that it is essential that the Ryan White program continues to be funded. A majority of those relying on the Ryan White program have insurance coverage, which suggests that Ryan White plays a fundamental role in the accessibility of high cost HIV medication and the range of services essential to engagement in medical treatment and adherence to medication (The Kaiser Family Foundation 2013). Importantly, the support provided by Ryan White funds has been related to viral suppression and to decrease in HIV incidence (The Kaiser Family Foundation 2013). Importantly, as the ACA is going into effect, the National HIV/AIDS Strategy has also been released. The National HIV/AIDS Strategy is the first comprehensive, National HIV/AIDS strategy in the U.S. (The Kaiser Family Foundation 2013). In order to successfully meet the priority goals of the National HIV/AIDS strategy, the continued funding of the Ryan White program in coordination with the ACA appears to be essential. The importance of ensuring continued funds for HIV/AIDS treatment is a clear priority as the American government repeatedly has approached shutdowns over budgetary debates and with the recent governmental shutdown surrounding the implementation of the ACA.

Importantly, Ryan White himself also gave a face to HIV/AIDS. Ryan White, a high school student with hemophilia, was infected with HIV in a manner that clearly defied the moralistic assumptions of HIV/AIDS. Giving a face to HIV that redefined the public discourse and imagery of HIV/AIDS was monumental in creating social change and providing treatment for PLWHA. This suggests that it is of the utmost importance for researchers to continue to work with professionals in industries with great public influence, such as the entertainment industry. Such collaborations can serve to change public conceptions of HIV/AIDS through the media and political influence. In addition, other historical human rights activists such as Nelson Mandela who publicly acknowledged that his son had died of AIDS, helped to give a face to HIV/AIDS and to move it from the realm of phantasm where secrecy and symbolism obscure and stigmatize the life conditions of PLWHA into the working world. Creative production has the potential to facilitate further HIV/AIDS activism. In order to facilitate the use of art, music, and writing to raise awareness of HIV/AIDS researchers are encouraged to further explore ways to reduce the fear of stigma and to protect PLWHA and those working to help them from legal and informal discrimination.

4.1.3 Experiments and Visions: Construction of Social Meaning

In this comparative biographical analysis, several unanticipated phenomena emerged. An unanticipated finding was the construction of social meaning in the form of the abstraction of visions and the construction of alternate realities. This was pronounced in Walter's construction of HIV as an experiment and of other participants in the Miami sample who described having visions. This allowed for an analysis of how people with HIV visualized their HIV, health, and life experiences in a symbolic way as grounded in personal biography. Furthermore, the construction of HIV as an experiment in the case of Walter initiated an analysis into the complex processes of acceptance versus denial of HIV and the deeply rooted nature of conceptions of HIV in personal history and cultural background. Importantly, transformative biographical processes such as those of creativity, entrepreneurship, innovation, and of spirituality emerged as unanticipated phenomena.

4.1.4 Intersectionality and HIV Experience

The intersection between ethnicity, sexuality, and HIV emerged as a central aspect of HIV experience. Discussions of racism were present in the story of Walter, an African American man interviewed in Frankfurt and among interviewees in the Miami sample. However, migrants in Germany did not explicitly discuss racism. It is not clear precisely what accounts for this difference. Perhaps, African American's experiences of racism are experienced in more active and rebellious ways because of civil rights activism and an awareness of a history of slavery, government exploitation, and racial inequality. The Hispanic participants tended to not discuss racism while the African American interviewees did describe racist attitudes in the United States. Perhaps in the local context of Miami, which is characterized by a large Hispanic population, Hispanics did not feel that racism was a major issue. However, additional research is needed which examines cross-cultural differences in the experience of racism in different nations, local contexts, and among different ethnic groups.

4.1.5   Creative Production and Entrepreneurship as Rebellion

Several biographical action process structures and transformative processes were identified. The development of creative potential was a driving force in people's lives, which helped them to overcome oppressive conditions related to marginalization and limited access to social and economic resources. The potential for change and transformative growth helped PLWHA to create new possibilities in their lives and to work to change the working world. Such transformational biographical processes have the potential for effective social change.

An important difference between the Frankfurt and the Miami samples was the emphasis on creative production, innovation, and entrepreneurship among the Miami sample as transformative biographical processes. While it is not possible to generalize, this difference may potentially be due to real cultural differences grounded in local and national context. The socio-political context of the U.S. has been described as having an overemphasis on individualism, materialism, consumerism, and inequality which can produce an enormous amount of strain on people to achieve financial goals (Merton 1938; Messner and Rosenfeld 2007). Merton (1938) argued that the differential access to legitimate means to the achievement of culturally defined goals can produce a sense of strain or anomie. Merton (1938) also posited that people can respond to strain in different modes of adaptation.

Merton's strain theory has been applied to criminal behavior but less is known about how adaptations to strain can drive entrepreneurship in contemporary American society. Innovation was defined by Merton (1938) as a mode of adaptation to strain, which involved the rejection of culturally acceptable means but acceptance of cultural goals. However, my results indicate that participants were engaged in adaptation by creating new enterprises that were not illegal. Engaging in creative production and entrepreneurship appeared to represent rebellion as described by Merton (1938). Entrepreneurship involved creating new means, which were innovative responses that created alternative opportunities to achieving new goals, and which were created based on life experience. For example, participants embarked on projects that were geared at informing the public discourse on HIV and had the potential to change socio-political and cultural context by raising awareness about HIV. These acts of creative production were processes wherein participants regained inspiration, purpose, and a sense of control over their lives. As Merton (1938) suggested, I found that these modes of adaptation to strain were rooted in personal experience and context as participants channeled their energies into HIV activism in order to help create HIV services to meet their needs that they felt were not fulfilled based on their personal experiences with HIV.

4.1.6   Financial Hardship and Medical Insurance Coverage

Financial stress and poverty were discussed in the Miami sample, suggesting that the strain in adaptation to the pursuit of economic security in the face of social inequality and limited social security was a major concern for the Miami participants. While this difference in poverty could be due to a sampling bias, estimates suggest that in the U.S. people with HIV disproportionately live in poverty (Karon et al. 2001; Holtgrave and Crosby 2003). In contrast, the Frankfurt sample did not discuss financial hardship or poverty. Interestingly, some interviewees actually expressed their concern for PLWHA in the U.S. because they felt that the American health care system did not provide the financial support necessary to cover medical care. The German health care system was discussed as vital to receiving quality health care and being able to afford HIV treatment, such as HIV medication and specialist care. Notably, David emphasized the multitude of problems that PLWHA have to face as he discussed the problems of insurance, medication, family conflict, culture, religion, homosexuality, and HIV that he felt were especially problematic for PLWHA in the U.S. who lack the insurance coverage of those in Germany.

The health care debate in America was discussed as obsolete. Some participants in the Frankfurt sample could not understand why the health care debate was still an issue and expressed a concern for PLWHA in the U.S., wondering how they could afford their medication in a context of limited insurance coverage. The former U.S. immigration ban for PLWHA was a barrier to HIV disclosure and health care access. The German mandatory dispersal of asylum seekers to remote reception centers was related to social isolation as demonstrated in the case of Rachel. The role of the German health care system in providing coverage of HIV medication and internationally focused specialist care was emphasized as integral to patients' health. In the U.S., participants had to remain in poverty in order to qualify for drug assistance programs, which exposed them to additional stressors and perpetuated social inequality.

Accordingly, my results were consistent with previous medical sociological approaches to social stress. Specifically, I found that many participants had to contend with a constellation of stressors, which supports social stress theory where primary stressors in one area of life are posited to proliferate and intersect with other stressors, and where stressors are conceptualized as being rooted in social positions and resources (Turner et al. 1995; Pearlin et al. 2005). The more limited insurance coverage and restrictive eligibility requirements for medical coverage in the U.S. served to limit participants' opportunities and to increase exposure to stressful life conditions, such as poverty, problems with medication coverage, and continuity of care. My findings support the suggestions by stress researchers that when examining social stress, historical time and place need to be considered and that lives are interdependent and should be examined as coherent life stories (Elder et al. 1996). My results are supported by other biographical research such as that of Ciambrone (2001), who found that HIV was initially experienced by HIV-positive women as biographically disruptive, but that other stressful life experiences, such as violence, mother-child separation, and drug use were discussed as more disruptive than HIV. Thus, my results are consistent with prior research and emphasized the multidimensionality of stress and life experience.

The high cost of HIV medication was not discussed as stressful for the Frankfurt sample. However, for participants in Miami, medication cost and limited health insurance coverage was a constant struggle. Participants in Miami discussed major disruptions in their continuity of care and quality of life due to their insurance coverage, which forced them to change doctors more often and to limit their incomes so that they could be eligible for Medicaid and drug assistance programs. Financial freedom and resources were discussed as important in facilitating their decision and ability to take action and taking control of their HIV. Insurance policy was linked to personal experience in biographical action, affecting feelings of control and stability. The Ryan White Foundation was described as helping participants to afford their medical treatment. Expansion of existing medical coverage to cover long-term care with a broad range of medical specialists and treatment centers could encourage patients to continue treatment with medical professionals of their preference instead of being forced by financial pressures to change their medical treatment. The disability and low-income requirements for medical coverage were also problematic and could contribute to the perpetuation of social disadvantage and serve as a barrier to upward social mobility. The implications of these limitations of American health care policy are further discussed in the policy implication section.

4.1.7   Compassionate Love and Social Support

The action process structure of compassionate love and social support in relations of care was discussed in both samples. Giving and receiving compassionate love was a biographical action process structure emergent on the relational level of social experience. Other research indicates that positive life change can involve compassionate love and can improve well-being among people with HIV (Lutz et al. 2011). Compassionate love is a concept recently elaborated by Underwood (2008) which involves: freedom of choice, cognitive understanding, value-empowerment, openness and receptivity, response of the heart, concern, and action. A prominent Harvard Sociologist Pitirim Sorokin, who was a mentor of Robert Merton, and who Merton credited for inspiring him to pursue sociology focused on love in his research but criticisms of the scientific study of love contributed to a turn away from sociological studies of love in subsequent years (Oman 2010; Sorokin 2002). Compassionate love is a concept that is not restricted to a psychological analysis and which has shown promise as a focus of sociological work (Oman 2010). In my study, compassionate love was discussed as being both given and received between participants and their children, intimate partners, and other close relations. Compassionate love invoked elements of generativity because relationships of care were an interchange, which facilitated personal growth and change and held a transformative potential for PLWHA. Additional research using a sociological framework could help to further develop the relationships between compassionate love and caregiving.

Social support also emerged as important to biographical action processes. Compassionate love can be viewed as distinct from social support because compassionate love involves a deep and loving commitment to care. Compassionate love involves a deep emotional and personal connection to others and to the self and can form the basis of meaningful social bonds, reducing social isolation and anomie. Additional research is encouraged to further develop the concepts of compassionate love and social support. However, for purposes of the current study, the identification of compassionate love and social support as key to human action was a contribution to the existing research on HIV and coping in a sociological framework.

As anticipated, both emotional and instrumental social support were related to personal growth and coping in the face of HIV. Social support was an important resource that mitigated the negative impact of HIV and other stressful life experiences on well-being. Social support was associated with an increased access to other resources including social capital, psychosocial resources such as sense of control and self-esteem, and economic resources. These resources were related to social networks. This is consistent with Bourdieu's definition social capital as actual or potential resources connected to social networks (Bourdieu 1985). Social networks and social capital were closely related and access to social networks and their corresponding resources was associated with group membership and sense of belonging.

These findings suggest that relations of care and resources linked to social networks are important in facilitating an escape from the trajectory of suffering of HIV. Similar to prior research, relations of care between participants and their children were reported as important to coping with HIV in both samples and among both men and women (Wilson 2007). Having children was important to participants because children provided them with a purpose to live, a sense of normality, and a sense of belonging and love. Some participants had their children before their HIV diagnosis while others had their children after diagnosis. The discussions of pregnancy after HIV diagnosis emphasized the importance of the dissemination of information to HIV patients regarding the possibility to have HIV-negative children despite their diagnosis and informing them of the appropriate prenatal and birthing medical care to prevent mother-to-child HIV transmission. Prior research suggests that HIV-positive mothers have to contend with issues of stigma and their roles as mothers can be made especially stressful by their HIV diagnosis (Wilson 2007). Furthermore, for those who had their children prior to HIV diagnosis, counseling services helped parents negotiate decisions related to their disclosure to their children and to cope with their fears of secondary stigma to their families. Counseling and support services can help PLWHA and their families to cope with HIV in a collective and supportive way.

Furthermore, involvement in support groups was reported as important in both samples and as providing participants with a sense of belonging, information about HIV, and increasing their social networks and resources. However, issues in seeking support services and utilization emerged in both samples. Interviewees explained how group identification and a sense of belonging were related to their decision to be members of support groups. When support groups were not felt to be consistent with one's identity or social position, support groups were not utilized. Barriers to social support service utilization included group identification, proximity to support services, procedural issues of timing, and fear of stigma. Importantly, involvement in support groups helped people to overcome their fears of stigma and to seek additional HIV services. However, fear of stigma was often a barrier to participation in support groups and this dialectic between stigma and support needed to be negotiated.

4.1.8   Spirituality and Religion

Notably, spirituality emerged as an especially important transformative biographical process structure in the Miami sample. The emphasis on spirituality and religion may have been due to the research design which involved semi-structured interviews that focused on spirituality and religion. Discussions of conceptions of sin and sexuality were also discussed by some of the gay men in the Frankfurt sample, but they did not elaborate in as much detail about the relationships between religion, spirituality, and sexuality as those in the Miami sample. Overcoming spiritual struggles was often reported as helping participants to come to terms with their HIV, their sexuality, and to stop risky behavior, such as unsafe sex and drug use. Interestingly, Ironson et al. (2011) found that among people living with HIV, having a view of God as benevolent and forgiving versus judgmental and punishing predicted disease progression. Shifts in conceptions of religion and positive spiritual growth involving positive views and relationships to the spiritual can be an integral aspect of meaning making and integration of HIV into biography.

Similar to other biographical research on HIV, religious experiences grounded in biography were related to meaning making and coping in my study (Jacobson et al. 2006). Because spirituality and religion can be related to coping and because coping has been found to be associated with health behaviors, such as medication adherence, health care utilization, treatment retention, and quality of life, research focusing on religious and spiritual aspects of coping can have implications for health (Blashill et al. 2011). Indeed, previous research has found that increases in spirituality and religiousness can occur after HIV diagnosis, and that increases in spirituality/religiousness predict disease progression, and can be related to cessation of destructive behavior such as drug use (Ironson et al. 2006; Kremer et al. 2009).

Spirituality was especially important for the gay men interviewed. In this study, some of these men reported experiencing abuse by priests in their childhood or adolescence and had to come to terms with their experience of abuse. Also, because of religious doctrines that condemn gay sexuality, gay men had to negotiate feelings of being unworthy of the spiritual and of reconciling their sexualities with their own personal relationships to the spiritual. Also, because HIV was tied to conceptions of deviant sexual behavior, women with histories of risky sexual behavior felt that they had to reconcile their sexual histories with the religious judgment by others of their lifestyles and identities as inherently sinful and deviant. Participants with contested statuses of being gay, drug users, or sexually deviant had to struggle to reframing their social experiences in a manner which allowed for a meaningful relationship with the spiritual and that reinvented their personal conceptions of the meanings of religion, sin, and their personal histories.

In the Miami sample, stigma was discussed in the context of religion, which could reflect the influence of the semi-structured interview format on interviewees' reconstruction of their life experiences because the interviews focused on religion and spirituality. However, the discussion of stigma in religious context was useful in examining the moral discourse of religious doctrines in relation to conceptions of HIV, sin, deviant behavior, and sexuality that may have otherwise not have been as pronounced. The discussion of stigma in religious context highlighted the role of moral discourse rooted in personal and collective culture in creating and maintaining HIV stigma. The conceptions of moral behavior and of sin versus morality, which form a major basis of religious doctrines, contribute to HIV stigma by condemning behavior and lifestyles that are not consistent with religious doctrines of righteousness. The association of HIV with contested or marginalized social status serves to stigmatize not only those whose backgrounds are consistent with HIV stereotypes, such as gay man, drug users, and those with risky sexual histories, but also serves to damage the legitimacy of PLWHA whose personal histories and social status are not consistent with these negative stereotypes. Future research is encouraged to further examine the ongoing interplay between negative HIV-related stereotypes and the perpetuation of stigma. Interviews with religious and community leaders and people without HIV could help to generate insights into the perpetuation of stigma as it relates to religious and moral discourse.

My analysis suggests that HIV presented a profound existential threat upon diagnosis among PLWHA. Accordingly, HIV could pose a disturbance of routine existence and social reality for people without HIV, which could threaten people's notions of their own mortality. The moral discourse surrounding HIV could be rooted in a primordial fear of death, which is layered beneath a dynamic interplay of social meanings and imagery. Stigma could represent a distancing response from this threat to the self and to mortality and may even be hidden from the awareness of those with stigmatizing attitudes and behavior. Supportive of this proposition, prior research indicates that perceptions of dangerousness and preferences for social distance predict public support of social control (Mossakowski et al. 2011). Stigma is a multi-dimensional concept that requires continued research from multiple perspectives of the public and the stigmatized.

Stigma emerged as a problematic and enduring challenge for PLWHA in both Miami and Frankfurt. Consistent with previous studies, participants described anticipation and internalization or felt stigma, experienced stigma, and secondary stigma or the proliferation of stigma to intimate others in this study (Wilson 2007; Carricaburu and Pierret 1995). Participants experienced stigma from their family members, intimate partners, friends, and in the workplace. Fear of experiencing stigma in the occupational sphere was especially pronounced in the Frankfurt sample and both samples expressed a fear of rejection in intimate relationships and saw their HIV as a barrier to finding and maintaining a romantic partnership.

4.1.9   Stigma and Appearance

Importantly, in both samples the importance of the body and appearance in relation to stigma was emphasized. Participants who experienced alterations to their appearance often felt exposed to stigma. Appearance was discussed as a distinguishing factor between those who experienced stigma versus those who did not. Bodily markers of illness such as extreme thinness or wasting served as symbolic markers of illness. Medication use can further problematize issues related to appearance because prior studies demonstrate that antiretroviral therapy can contribute to conditions such lipodystrophy, which alter the body's appearance by producing extreme weight loss (lipoatrophy) or weight gain (hyperadiposity) (Collins et al. 2000; Schwenk et al. 2000). Prior studies indicate that experiencing lipodystrophy and other side effects of HIV medication are related to emotional difficulties in social and sexual relations, and are related to demoralization and to forced disclosure (Collins et al. 2000; Kremer et al. 2009). In my analysis, participants emphasized the role of the visibility of HIV in contributing to verbal stigma where others gossiped about their health. This gossip contributed to a great deal of stress, social withdrawal, and was disruptive to social relationships. Participants valued maintaining an attractive and healthy appearance and minor cosmetic procedures emerged as a means of regaining a healthy body image and of protecting against stigma.

4.2   Limitations

This project has several limitations which should be acknowledged. First, I did not design or conduct the interviews among the Miami sample. The Miami sample was not recruited on-site at a treatment facility and interviewees visited a university research center to participate in the Miami study. Also, the interview structure was semi-structured and not open-ended for the Miami sample. However, interviewees were interviewed at multiple time points and also completed essays, questionnaires, and their transcripts contained case notes for subsequent time points. This additional data helped me to reconstruct interviewees' narratives.

The modes of recruitment and location site of the interviews could have created sampling bias in both samples. For example, the high monetary compensation for participation in the Miami study could have encouraged more socioeconomically disadvantaged participants to agree to the Miami study. In contrast, all of the participants in the Frankfurt sample were in treatment. The participants in the Frankfurt sample were recruited on-site and the interview setting was an international HIV clinic where participants were receiving treatment. However, the differences in the samples provided an opportunity to study PLWHA from a broad range of backgrounds. The comparison of the interviews in Frankfurt and Miami allowed for a cross-cultural comparison that took cultural context and social policy related to health care and immigration law into account.

Immigration was discussed among the Frankfurt sample but experiences with immigration were not discussed in the Miami interviews. However, Miami is a major metropolitan area characterized by high levels of immigration (Department of Homeland Security 2009b; The Brookings Institute 2004). Perhaps poverty was a more central concern for the Miami sample in a context of lacking financial support for optimal HIV treatment in a highly gentrified, major city in America. Similar to recent estimates, which indicate that rates of HIV prevalence are higher among those living in poverty and that disadvantaged groups have disproportionate rates of HIV infection, poverty and social inequality were emphasized by participants in the Miami sample (Denning 2010). The economic concerns discussed by participants could have reflected the sociocultural context Miami, which is an area characterized by high levels of income inequality and residential segregation (Pew 2012).

The relationship between poverty and HIV emphasizes the importance of cost-reduction of HIV treatment for patients. Insurance coverage for HIV medication was problematic due to the high cost of medication and limited coverage among the Miami sample. Access to medical treatment and insurance coverage to cover the cost of HIV treatment was discussed as a major benefit of living in Germany. Having to pay out of pocket expenses for HIV treatment was felt to be a major limitation to maintaining a standard of living above the poverty level and being able to continue HIV treatment. The different socio-cultural contexts involving health insurance policy and social inequality were intertwined with trajectories of suffering and were contextual conditions of participants' trajectories of suffering. Restrictions in spatial and economic freedom appeared to have a major impact of coping with HIV.

Potentially due to the different interview types, stigma was discussed more often in a religious context in the Miami sample than in the Frankfurt interviews. Religion and spirituality were emphasized more in the Miami interviewees as interviewers asked questions about religion and spirituality and probed about these topics. The difference in interview type demonstrates the influence of research design and methodology on research findings. Interview designs that involve an open question format may be helpful in order to not lead interviewees away from themes that could be important to interviewees' narratives. For example, neighborhood conditions such as neighborhood poverty, racial segregation, and dangerous housing conditions were mentioned in the Miami interviews but the structure of the interviews often guided participants away from a deeper discussion of neighborhood context.

A limitation of the interviews I designed and implemented in Frankfurt was that they were restricted to English-speaking patients at the clinic. However, my sample was diverse and included both men and women native to Germany and migrants from other nations. The medical staff was fluent in English due to the international nature of the clinic, which made communication effective with staff and many of the patients could speak English at an adequate or high language proficiency level.

Another limitation was that none of the interviewees were self-reported injection drug users. Recruiting interviewees on-site may have not allowed for the inclusion of those who were more disadvantaged, engaged in high risk lifestyles, or were transient. Also, the Miami sample was screened for current injection drug use and therefore self-reported injected drug users were not included in the Miami sample. The exclusion was due to the principal investigator's collection of biomarkers of CD4 cell-count, viral load, and stress hormones, which could be affected by drug use. Future studies are encouraged to utilize multiple recruitment sites for interviews and to include injection drug users.

Despite this limitation, a major strength of on-site recruitment was my access to the context of the medical treatment center where participants were seeking care. The clinic provided a support group "Helping Hand" where medical staff referred their high risk patients for support, information about HIV, and which provided group activities. This allowed for an analysis of the effectiveness of Helping Hand and how this service could be a helpful model for future on-site support programs. Helping Hand was a promising program that has received attention from the General U.S. Consulate in Frankfurt and which has policy implications for effective health care coordination of essential services. While my findings are not generalizable to all PLWHA, an advantage of this biographical analysis was theoretical elaboration grounded in personal and collective histories in a cross-cultural context.

4.3   Policy Implications

This study has important policy implications for health care. The comparison of different health care contexts was rooted in broader policy decisions and political discourse. The financial problems in obtaining adequate medical coverage were real concerns related to American health care policy. The findings presented in this manuscript suggest that the requirements for eligibility for AIDS Drug Assistance Programs (ADAPs) and Medicaid can be problematic. These findings correspond to prior research which suggests that eligibility for antiretroviral treatment was related to continuity of care among HIV patients (Torian and Wiewel 2011). At the time of the Miami interview completion, the ACA had not yet gone into effect. Therefore, problems related to being refused medical insurance due to HIV as a pre-existing condition and the requirement to be on disability to receive support for HIV treatment may be less pronounced in light of recent policy change. However, the ACA still requires a low-income requirement for government assistance to pay for medical care. This low-income requirement was problematic because it prevented some participants from continuing full-time employment and may have prevented those in poverty from being motivated and able to obtain higher-income employment.

The original title of title of the ACA was the "Patient Protection and Affordable Care Act". While this change appears to be subtle, it also carries significance to public discourse surrounding health care in the United States. It is possible that terminology used to frame policy change can have implications to the construction of meaning and public understanding of this policy change. Specifically, how the

ACA is being received by the American public could be influenced by removing the "patient protection" wording because taking out patient protection removes from public discourse the role of the ACA initiative to protect human rights. In order for the successful implementation of a program it must be well-received by the target population. When the implementation of health care policy is not tailored to the cultural context of American ideological beliefs and the American public's concerns it runs the risk of not being accepted by its intended recipients of care.

Therefore, it is critical to understand American public attitudes towards health care because a lack of information about the policy change and deeply-rooted suspicions of governmental control and fears of taxation could contribute to a resistance to universal health care coverage thus undermining the public's interests. Without awareness of specific policy measures, and with a lack of trusting and collaborative relationships between government and civil society, there could be a collective reversal of agency where people take actions against their own benefit. Through effective communication and collaboration a successful negotiation of health care policy concerns could be facilitated. In this study, some participants described lacking information about HIV at their diagnosis and struggled with the acceptance of HIV. HIV prevention and treatment programs should be mainstreamed into social policy so that vulnerable populations do not have limited access and reduced utilization of health care because of discrimination and fear of stigma.

It is also important to note that the current enormous health care policy shift is not occurring in a social vacuum. Rather, the ACA is being implemented in a context of an ongoing commodification of health care and ideological beliefs that center on individual liberty and a free market economic system. The ongoing history of the commodification of health care in the United States may continue to be a major challenge to effective health care reform as various stakeholders lobby for their interests in a free market. While beyond the scope of the current study, it appears that it is of the utmost importance to increase effective communication between the insurance companies, pharmaceutical and medical technology industries, government, physicians, and patients in their respective arenas. Through open communication of these actors' concerns and interests, policies can be developed with an evidence-based approach in order to ensure quality health care and to reduce political conflict.

Collaborative relationships with pharmaceutical companies manufacturing HIV medication could contribute to the development of HIV services. For example, Helping Hand was funded by the city of Frankfurt and pharmaceutical companies. My results indicate that Helping Hand was a successful intervention improving the psychosocial functioning of patients, reducing social isolation, and helped members to develop a sense of belonging and to negotiate stigma. Therefore, developing positive relationships between medical facilities and pharmaceutical companies with a patient-centered approach focused on the provision of quality medical care could improve health care. By working in a collaborative spirit of mutual interest focused on improving health services for patients, Helping Hand provided a useful model for future HIV interventions. Evidence-based research informed by all respective parties in health care could help to increase our knowledge of effective health care policy. A patient-centered approach to health care can be used to further inform the development and design of future programs for HIV-positive patients.

The policy implications of this study highlight the importance of the interdependence of health and immigration policy. This analysis emphasized the importance of immigration policy in the lives of PLWHA. In Germany, regulations designed to cut the cost of immigration by placing asylum seekers in specific locations upon their arrival can serve to socially and spatially isolate migrants, and can be especially problematic for asylum seekers with HIV who are in need of the support of their families and friends and of health care professionals (Boswell 2003). Spatial dislocation from HIV treatment centers and support services could be a barrier to service utilization and continuity of care. Specialization of medical care was positively valued by participants and access to HIV specialists was an important aspect of their HIV treatment. For example, participants in the Frankfurt sample often framed their current treatment at the HIV clinic in positive light in comparison to medical treatment they had received from general practitioners or other hospitals and emphasized the quality of care and medical knowledge of the physicians at the HIV clinic. Participants in the Miami sample also emphasized the importance of receiving treatment from HIV specialists who were aware of state of the art treatment and research in the field of HIV.

U.S. immigration law until recently had a ban on immigration for people with HIV (Brown and Cetron 2011). Recently, HIV has been removed from the Center for Disease Control's (CDC) list of communicable diseases, which was meant reduce barriers to entry and stay for PLWHA (Brown and Cetron 2011). However, at the time of the interviews, this ban was not yet lifted. My analysis suggests that immigration and health care policy are interrelated and each should be taken into context when designing and implementing programs. For example, immigration policies that encourage referrals to HIV testing, treatment, and support centers could help people with HIV navigate the health care system. International health care centers such as the university clinic and the support service Helping Hand can provide a useful framework for the development of successful HIV treatment centers. The coordination of immigration and health care systems can be further informed by additional research using the biographical approach to understand how these policies are experienced as institutional channels of illness experience by patients and practitioners and which cannot be divorced from cultural context. Biographical policy analysis applied to the exploration of how people experience and deal with the policies that impact their lives, and which can help to develop an understanding of how health practitioners reflect on their own practices and the institutions in which they work, could help to inform HIV policy (Dausein et al. 2008).

My findings suggest that cultural context is important because beliefs grounded in cultural context intersected in participants' meaning making of HIV and can affect coping, chronic disease management, and health behaviors. Furthermore, consistent with other studies, I found that stigma was a major barrier to service utilization (Varas-Díaz et al. 2005; Mahajan 2008). Stigma was a challenge for participants in both samples. Previous research emphasizes the negative impact of stigma on sexual risk behavior such as condom use, service utilization, and HIV testing (Kalichman and Simbayi 2003; Mahajan et al. 2008; Varas-Díaz et al. 2005; Ross et al. 2013). Engagement in support programs such as Helping Hand could help to reduce feelings of stigma and encourage participation in health care services and integration into a supportive, empowered community. Overcoming stigma could help to facilitate disclosure of HIV, increase access to social resources and a collective identity, and allow for the shift from a marginalized identity to an empowered, project identity, which could allow for change in public discourse surrounding HIV (Castells 1997; Parker and Aggleton 2003). However, being open about HIV often came at a great personal cost, with participants losing their careers, social standing, and relationships. Therefore, policies aimed at legally prohibiting the discrimination of PLWHA could help to protect PLWHA from these losses and to encourage their openness about HIV.

Interventions designed to reduce stigma and to help patients cope with the stress of discrimination are needed. Legal protections for vulnerable populations are necessary to ensure the protection of human rights. Furthermore, educational efforts about HIV should be mainstreamed into broader educational systems. In this way, the broader community can be familiarized with HIV at a larger scale and earlier in the life course. Furthermore, stigma can proliferate to the families and communities of those living with HIV/AIDS and therefore policies to reduce stigma should be multifaceted and targeted to families and communities (Cluver et al. 2008). Interventions that provide both information about the mode of HIV transmission and that also give a face to HIV could be effective in reducing stigma. As long as HIV remains faceless it lacks representation and is subject to negative, dehumanizing stereotypes that can foster social distance. Interventions to reduce stigma must contend with the emotional and moralistic aspects of stigma. A possibility for such programs could involve the use of personal stories, visual art, film, and music to facilitate awareness of HIV and a sense of human connection and compassion with others.

Bibliography

Abali, O.S. (2009): *German Public Opinion on Immigration and Integration.* Washington, DC.
Abraído-Lanza, A.F., Guier, C. and Colón, R.M. (1998): Psychological Thriving Among Latinas With Chronic Illness. *Journal of Social Issues,* 54: 405–424. doi: 10.1111/j.1540-4560.1998.tb01227.x
Anant, S.S. (1966): The Need to Belong. Canada's *Mental Health,* 14: 21-27.
Antoni, M.H., Cruess, D.G., Cruess, S., Lutgendorf, S., Kumar, M., Ironson, G., Klimas, N., Fletcher, M.A., Schneiderman, N. (2000): Cognitive-Behavioral Stress Management Intervention Effects on Anxiety, 24-Hr Urinary Norepinephrine Output, and T-Cytotoxic/Suppressor Cells Over Time Among Symptomatic HIV-Infected Gay Men. *Journal of Consulting and Clinical Psychology* 68: 31-45.
Antoni, M.H., Baggett, L., Ironson, G., LaPerriere, A., August, S., Klimas, N. (1991): Cognitive-Behavioral Stress Management Intervention Buffers Distress Responses and Immunologic Changes Following Notification of HIV-1 Seropositivity. *Journal of Consulting and Clinical Psychology,* 59: 906-915.
Aneshensel, C.S. (1992): Social Stress: Theory and Research. *Annual Review of Sociology* 18:15-38.
Antiretroviral Therapy Cohort Collaboration (2008): Life expectancy of individuals on combination antiretroviral therapy in high-income countries: a collaborative analysis of 14 cohort studies. *Lancet* 372: 293-239.
Apitzsch, U., Siouti, I. (2007): Biographical Analysis as an interdisciplinary research perspective in Migration Studies. Accessed online January 1st 2013.
Apitzsch, U., Inowlocki, L. (2000): Biographical analysis. A German's School? In: Chamberlayne, P., Bornat, J., Wengraf, T. (Hg.): *The Turn to Biographical Methods in Social Sciences. Comparative Issues and Examples.* London, S. 53-70.
AVERT (2010): HIV & AIDS Stigma and Discrimination. http://www.avert.org/hiv-aids-stigma.htm. *Accessed May 20th 2010.*
Baron, R.M., Kenny, D.A. (1986): The Moderator-Mediator Variable Distinction in Social Psychological Research: Conceptual, Strategic, and Statistical Considerations. *Journal of Personality and Social Psychology* 51: 1173-1182.
Bayor, R.H. (ed.)(2003): Race and Ethnicity in America: A concise history. New York.
Bätzing-Feigenbaum, J., Loschen, S., Gohlke-Micknis, S., Zimmermann, R., Herrmann, A., Kamga Wambo, O., Kücherer, C., Hamouda, O. (2008): Country-wide HIV Incidence Study Complementing HIV Surveillance in Germany. *Eurosurveillance,* 13: 1-4.
Boswell, C. (2003): Burden-Sharing in the European Union: Lessons from the German and UK Experience. *Journal of Refugee Studies,* 16: 316-335.
Berger, P.L., Luckmann, T. (1966): *The Social Construction of Reality : A Treatise in the Sociology of Knowledge.* London.
Bergson, H. (1922) : *Durée et simultanéité : à propos de la théorie d'Einstein.* Paris. (English Translation 1935: Duration and Simultaneity, trans. B.A. Audra and C. Brereton with the assistance of W.H. Carter, London.
Bertaux, D. (2003): The Usefulness of Life Stories for a Realist and Meaningful Sociology. In: Humphrey, R., Miller, R., Zdravomyslova, E. (eds.): *Biographical Research in Eastern Europe: Altered lives and broken biographies.* Hampshire, p. 39-52.

Bertaux, D., Kohli, M. (1984): The Life Story Approach: A Continental View. *Annual Review of Sociology* 10: 215-237.

Betts, S., Griffiths, A., Schütze, F., Straus, P. (2004): Biographical Counseling: An Introduction. *European Studies on Inequalities and Social Cohesion*, p. 5-58.

Billings, D.W., Folkman, S., Acree, M.M., Moskowitz, J.T. (2000): Coping and Physical Health During Caregiving: The Roles of Positive and Negative Affect. *Journal of Personality and Social Psychology* 79:131-142.

Bing, E.G., Burnam, A., Longshore, D., Fleishman, J.A., Sherbourne, C.D., London, A.S., Turner, B.J., Eggan, F., Beckman, R., Vitiello, B., Morton, S.C., Orlando, M., Bozzette, S.A., Ortiz-Barron, L., Shapiro, M. (2001): Psychiatric Disorders and Drug Use among Human Immunodeficiency Virus–Infected Adults in the United States. *Archives of General Psychiatry*, 58: 721-728.

Blankenship, K.M. (1998): A Race, Class, and Gender Analysis of Thriving. *Journal of Social Issues*, 54: 393-404.

Blascovich, J., Spencer, S.J., Quinn, D., Steele, C. (2001): African Americans and High Blood Pressure: The Role of Stereotype Threat. *Psychological Science* 12: 225-229.

Blashill, A.J., Perry, N., Safren, S.A. (2011): Mental Health: A Focus on Stress, Coping, and Mental Illness as it Relates to Treatment Retention, Adherence, and Other Health Outcomes. *Current HIV/AIDS Reports*, 8: 215-222.

Blumer, H. (1969): *Symbolic Interactionism: Perspective and Method*. Berkeley.

Boyes, M.E., Cluver, L.D. (2013): Relationships amongst HIV/AIDS-orphanhood, stigma, and symptoms of anxiety and depression in South African youth: A longitudinal investigation using a path analysis framework. Clinical Psychological Science, 1 (3), 323-330.

Bourdieu, P. (1985): *The Forms of Capital*. In: Richardson, J.G. (ed.): Handbook of Theory and Research for the Sociology of Education. New York, pp. 241-58.

Bovier, P.A., Chamot, E., Perneger, T.V. (2004): Perceived stress, internal resources, and social support as determinants of mental health among young adults. *Quality of Life Research,* 13: 161-170.

Burke, P.J. (1991): Identity Processes and Social Stress. *American Sociological Review*, 56: 836-849.

Burke, P.J. (2007): Identity Control Theory. In: Ritzer, G. (ed.): *Blackwell Encyclopedia of Sociology*. Oxford.

Bury, M. (1982): Chronic Illness as Biographical Disruption. *Sociology of Health and Illness*, 4: 167-182.

Brown, Clive M., and Martin S. Cetron (2011): Crossing Borders: One World, Global Health. *Clinical Infectious Diseases,* 53: September. http://cid.oxfordjournals.org/. Accessed online January 29th, 2012.

Brown, L., Macintyre, K., Trujillo L. (2003): Interventions to Reduce HIV/AIDS Stigma: What Have We Learned? *AIDS Education and Prevention* 15: 49-69.

Burchardt, M. (2010): 'Life in Brackets': Biographical Uncertainties of HIV-Positive Women in South Africa. *Forum: Qualitative Social Research,* 11: 1-18.

Cao, X., Sullivan, S.G., Xu, J., Wu, Z., and the China CIRPA Project 2 Team (2006): Understanding HIV-Related Stigma and Discrimination in a "Blameless" Population. *AIDS Education and Prevention* 18: 518-528.

Capitanio, J.P., Abel, K., Mendoza, S.P., Blozis, S.A., McChesney, M.B., Cole, S.W., Mason, W.A. (2008): Personality and serotonin transporter genotype interact with social context to affect immunity and viral set-point in simian immunodeficiency virus disease. *Brain, Behavior, and Immunity*, 22: 676-689.

Carricaburu, D., Pierret, J. (1995): From biographical disruption to biographical reinforcement: the case of HIV-positive men. *Sociology of Health & Illness,* 17: 65-88.

Castells, M. (1997): *The Power of Identity*. Oxford.

Centers for Disease Control and Prevention. *HIV Surveillance Report, 2010*; vol. 22. http://www.cdc.gov/hiv/topics/surveillance/resources/reports/. Published March 2012. Accessed [February 7th, 2013].

Chamberlayne, P., Bornat, J., Wengraf, T. (2000): *The Turn to Biographical Methods in Social Sciences. Comparative Issues and Examples.* London.

Chanfrault-Duchet, M.F. (1995): Biographical Research in Former West Germany. *Current Sociology* 43: 209-219.

Charmaz, K. (1999): Stories of Suffering: Subjective Tales and Research Narrative. *Qualitative Health Research*, 9: 362-382.

Charmaz, K. (1995): The Body, Identity, and Self: Adapting to Impairment. *The Sociological Quarterly,* 36: 657-680.

Charmaz, K. (1991): *Good Days, Bad Days: The Self in Chronic Illness.* New Brunswick, NJ.

Charmaz, K. (1983): Loss of Self: A Fundamental Form of Suffering in the Chronically Ill. *Sociology of Health and Illness,* 5: 168-95.

Ciambrone, D. (2001): Illness and other assaults on the self: the relative impact of HIV/AIDS on women's lives. *Sociology of Health and Illness,* 23: 517-540.

Cluver, Lucie, Frances Gardner, D., Operario, D. (2008): Effects of Stigma on the Mental Health of Adolescents Orphaned by AIDS. *Journal of Adolescent Health,* 42: 410-417.

Collins E., Wagner, C., Walmsley, S. (2000): Psychosocial impact of the lipodystrophy syndrome in HIV infection. *The AIDS Reader,* 10: 546-550.

Cooley, C.H. (1902): *Human Nature and the Social Order.* New York.

Corbin, J., Strauss, A. (2007): *Basics of Qualitative Research: Techniques and Procedures for Developing Grounded Theory.* 3rd edition, Thousand Oaks.

Corbin, J., Strauss; A. (1990): Grounded Theory Research: Procedures, Canons and Evaluative Criteria. *Zeitschrift fuur Soziologie,* 19(6): 418-427.

Corbin, J., Strauss, A..L. (1988): *Unending Work and Care: Managing Chronic Illness at Home.* San Francisco.

Corrigan, P., Markowitz, F.E., Watson, A., Rowan, D., Kubiak, M.A. (2003): An Attribution Model of Public Discrimination Towards Persons with Mental Illness. *Journal of Health and Social Behavior* 44: 162-179.

Crocker, J., Major, B. (1989): Social stigma and self-esteem: The self-protective properties of stigma. *Psychological Review, 96,* 608-630.

Dausien, B., Hanses, A., Inowlocki, L., Riemann, G. (2008): The Analysis of Professional Practice, the Self-Reflection of Practitioners, and their Way of Doing Things. Resources of Biography Analysis and Other Interpretative Approaches. Forum: Qualitative Social Research, 9. www.qualitative-research.net/index.php/fqs/rt/printerFriendly/312/685. Accessed online April 4th, 2013.

Del Amo, J., Erwin, J., Fenton, K., Gray, K. (2001): AIDS & Mobility: Looking to the Future. Report Commisioned by the European Project AIDS & Mobility (NIGZ).

Denning P., DiNenno E. (2010): Communities in crisis: is there a generalized HIV epidemic in impoverished urban areas of the United States. Abstract WEPDD101. Presented at: XVIII International AIDS Conference, July 18-23, 2010, Vienna, Austria.

Department of Homeland Security (2012a): Annual Flow Report: U.S.: Legal Permanent Residents: 2011. http://www.dhs.gov/xlibrary/assets/statistics/publications/lpr_fr_2011.pdf. Accessed online February 7[th,] 2013.

Department of Homeland Security (2012b): Annual Flow Report: Refugees and Asylees: 2011. http://www.dhs.gov/xlibrary/assets/statistics/publications/ois_rfa_fr_2011.pdf. Accessed online February 7[th,] 2013.

Department of Homeland Security (2009): Fact Sheet: The Foreign-Born Component of the Uninsured Population. http://www.dhs.gov/immigrationstatistics. Accessed online February 7th, 2013.

Deutsche AIDS-Hilfe e.V. (2011): Drug Consumption Rooms in Germany: A Situational Assessment by the AK Konsumraum. Deutsche AIDS-Hilfe e.V. Berlin, September 2011.

Deutsche Gesellschaft für Internationale Zusammenarbeit (GIZ) GmbH (2012): The German Approach to HIV Mainstreaming: Effective Development Work in a Time of HIV. *German Health Practice Collection.*

Devine, P.G., Plant, E.A., Harrison, K. (1999): The Problem of "Us" Versus "Them" and AIDS Stigma. *American Behavioral Scientist* 42: 1212-1228.

Varas-Díaz, N., Serrano-García, I., Toro-Alfonso, J. (2005): AIDS-Related Stigma and Social Interaction: Puerto Ricans Living With HIV/AIDS. *Qualitative Health Research,* 2: 169-187.

Varas-Díaz, N., Toro-Alfonso, J. (2003): Incarnating Stigma: Visual Images of the Body with HIV/AIDS [59 paragraphs]. Forum Qualitative Sozialforschung / Forum: Qualitative Social Research [On-line Journal], 4(3). Available at: http://www.qualitative-research.net/fqstexte/3-03/3-03varastoro-e.htm [Date of access: January 1, 2013].

Dohrenwend, B.P., Levan, I., Shrout, P.E., Shwartz, S., Link, B.G., Skodol, A.E., Stueve, A. (1992): Socioeconomic Status and Psychiatric Diorders: The Causation-Selection Issue. *Science* 255: 946-952.

Dohrenwend, B.P., Dohrenwend, B.S. (1969): *Social Status and Psychological Disorder: A Causal Inquiry.* New York.

Elder, G., George, L., Shanahan, M. (1996): Psychosocial Stress Over the Life Course. In: Kaplan, H.A. (ed.): *Psychosocial Stress: Perspectives of Structure, Theory, Lifecourse, and Methods.* San Diego, pp. 247-291.

Emerson, R.M. (1976): Social Exchange Theory. *Annual Review of Sociology* 2: 335-362.

European Centre for Disease Prevention and Control/WHO Regional Office for Europe (2011): HIV/AIDS surveillance in Europe 2010. Stockholm: European Centre for Disease Prevention and Control.

Falk, G. (2001): *Stigma: How we treat outsiders.* New York.

Fekete, E.M, Antoni, M.H., Lopez, C.R., Duran, R.E., Penedo, F.J., Bandiera, F.C., Fletcher, M.A., Klimas, N., Kumar, M., Schneiderman, N. (2009): Men's Serostatus Disclosure to Parents: Associations Among Social Support, Ethnicity, and Disease Status in Men Living with HIV. *Brain, Behavior, and Immunology* 23: 693-699.

Florida Department of Health (2009): Statistics: HIV/AIDS Statistics. http://www.careresource.org/hivaids/statistics/. Accessed online February 7th, 2013.

Freund, P.E.S., McGuire, M.B. (1991): *Health, Illness, and the Social Body: A Critical Sociology.* Englewood Cliffs, NJ.

Gächter, M., Savage, D.A., Torgler, B. (2009): The relationship between stress, strain and social capital. *Working Papers* from Faculty of Economics and Statistics, University of Innsbruck.

Gaines, S. (2009): *Fool's Paradise.* New York.

Geertz, C. (1973): *The interpretation of cultures: Selected essays.* New York.

Greene, K., Banerjee, S.C. (2006): Disease-Related Stigma: Comparing Predictors of AIDS and Cancer Stigma. *Journal of Homosexuality,* 50: 185-209.

Giddens, A. (1995; 1981): Agency, Instution, and Time-Space Analysis. In: McQuarie, D. (ed.): *Readings in Contemporary Sociological Theory: From Modernity to Post-Modernity.* Prentice Hall, pp. 335-343.

Glaser, B.G., Strauss, A.L. (1965): *Awareness of Dying.* New Brunswick, NJ.

Goffman, E. (1963): *Stigma: Notes on the Management of Spoiled Identity.* New Jersey.

Goffman, E. (1959): *The Presentation of Self in Everyday Life.* New York.

Goode, W.J. (1960): A Theory of Role Strain. *American Sociological Review,* 25: 483-496.

Gramling, R., Forsyth, C.J. (1987): Exploiting Stigma. *Sociological Forum* 2: 401-415.

Hall, H.I., Song, R., Rhodes, P., Prejean, J., Q, A., Lee, L.M., Karon, J., Brookmeyer, R., Kaplan, E.H., McKenna, M.T., Janssen, R.S. (2008): Estimation of HIV Incidence in the United States. *JAMA,* 300: 520-525.

Hansen, R. (2003): Migration to Europe since 1945: Its History and its Lessons. The Political Quarterely Publishing Co. Ltd. United Kingdom: Oxford, pp. 25-38.

Haug, W., Compton, P., Courbage, Y. (eds.)(2002): The demographic characteristics of immigrant populations. Council of Europe. *The Population Studies Series, 38.*

Hagerty, B.M.K., Lynch-Sauer, J., Patusky, K.L., Bouwsema, M., Collier, P. (1992): Sense of Belonging: A Vital Mental Health Concept. *Archives of Psychiatric Nursing,* 3: 172-177.

Herek, G.M. (1996): *AIDS and Stigma: A Conceptual Framework and Research Agenda.* The National Institute of Mental Health Research Workshop Final Report. Accessed online August 29th, 2012.

Herek, G.M. (1999): AIDS and Stigma. *American Behavorial Scientist* 42: 1106-1116.

Hogg, M.A., Terry, D.J., White, K.M. (1995): A Tale of Two Theories: A Critical Comparison of Identity Theory with Social Identity Theory. *Social Psychology Quarterly* 58: 255-269.

Holtgrave, D.R., Crosby, R.A. (2003): Social capital, poverty, and income inequality as predictors of gonorrhoea, syphilis, chlamydia and AIDS case rates in the United States. *Sexually Transmitted Infections,* 79: 62-64.

House, J.S., Kahn, R.L. (1985): Measures and Concepts of Social Support. In: Cohen, S., Syme, S.L. (eds.): *Social Support and Health.* Academic Press, p. 83-108.

Howard, J.A. (2000): Social Psychology of Identities. *Annual Review of Sociology* 26: 367-393.

Husserl, E. (1964): *Phenomenology of Internal Time Consciousness.* First edition. Editor: Heidegger, M. Translated by James S. Churchill. Indiana.

Husserl, E., Brough, J.B. (1991): *Collected Works: On the phenomenology of the consciousness of internal time (1893-1917).* Editor: John B. Brough. Translated by Brough, John Barnett. Berlin.

Idemudia, E.S., Matamela, N.A. (2012): The role of stigmas in mental health: A comparative study. *Curationis 35(1),* Art. #30, 8 pages. http://dx.doi.org/10.4102/curationis.v35i1.30.

International Organization for Migration (IOM). "Key issues on HIV, TB and international population mobility." September, 2007.

Ironson G., Stuetzle R., Ironson D., Balbin E., Kremer H., George A., Schneiderman N., Fletcher, M.A. (2011): View of God as benevolent and forgiving or punishing and judgmental predicts HIV disease progression. *Journal of Behavioral Medicine,* 34:414-25.

Ironson, G., Kremer, H. (2011): Coping, spirituality, and health in HIV. In: Folkman, S. (ed.): *The Oxford Handbook of Stress, Health, and Coping.* Oxford, p. 289-318.

Ironson, G., Kremer, H., Ironson, D. (2006): Spirituality, Spiritual Experiences, and Spiritual Transformations in the Face of HIV. In: Koss, J.D., Hefner, P. (eds.): *Spiritual Transformation and Healing,* 1st ed., Oxford, pp. 241-262.

Ironson, G., O'Cleirigh, C., Fletcher, M.A., Laurenceau, J.P., Balbin, E., Klimas, N. (2005): Psychosocial Factors Predict CD4 and Viral Load Change in Men and Women With Human Immunodeficiency Virus in the Era of Highly Active Antiretroviral Treatment. *Psychosomatic Medicine,* 67: 1013-1021.

Ironson, G., Friedman, A., Klimas, N., Antoni, M., Fletcher, M.A., Laperriere, A. (1994): Distress, Denial, and Low Adherence to Behavioral Interventions Predict Faster Disease Progression in Gay Men Infected with Human Immunodeficiency Virus. *International Journal of Behavioral Medicine* 1:90-105.

Jacobson, J.C. Jr., Luckhaupt, S.E., Delaney, S., Tsevat, J. (2006): Religio-Biography, Coping, and Meaning-Making Among Persons with HIV/AIDS. *Journal for the Scientific Study of Religion,* 45: 39-56.

Jacoby, A. (1994): Felt versus enacted stigma: a concept revisited: evidence from a study of people with epilepsy in remission. *Social Science and Medicine,* 38: 269-274.

Jones, C.P. (2000): Levels of Racism: A Theoretical Framework and a Gardener's Tale. *American Journal of Public Health,* 90: 1212-1215.

Jones, E., Farina, A., Hastorf, A., Markus, H., Miller, D.T., Scott, R. (1984): *Social Stigma: The Psychology of Marked Relationships.* New York.

The Kaiser Family Foundation (2013): Updating the Ryan White HIV/AIDS Program for a New Era: Key Issues and Questions for the Future. http://kaiserfamilyfoundation.files.wordpress.com/2013/04/8431.pdf. Accessed online December 19th, 2013.

The Kaiser Family Foundation (2012): An Update on the ACA & HIV: Medicaid Health Homes. http://kff.org/health-reform/fact-sheet/quick-take-an-update-on-the-aca/. Accessed online February 7th, 2012.

Kalichman, S.C., Simbayi, L.C. (2003): HIV testing attitudes, AIDS stigma, and voluntary HIV counselling and testing in a black township in Cape Town, South Africa. *Sexually Transmitted Infections,* 79:442-447.

Karon, J.M., Fleming, P.L., Steketee, R.W., De Cock, K.M. (2001): HIV in the United States at the Turn of the Century: An Epidemic in Transition. *American Journal of Public Health,* 91: 1060-1068.

Kelly, B., Raphael, B., Mudd, F., Percides, M., Kernutt, G., Burnett, P., Dunne, M., Burrows, G. (1998): Posttraumatic stress disorder in response to HIV infection. *General Hospital Psychiatry* 20: 345-352.

Kessler, R.C., Neighbors, H.W. (1986): A New Perspective on the Relationships among Social Race, Social Class, and Psychological Distress. *Journal of Health and Social Behavior.* 27: 107-115.

Kremer, H. (2012): USA: Banning People with HIV from Attending the AIDS 2012 Conference. http://www.opendemocracy.net/5050/heidemarie-f-kremer/usa-banning-people-with-hiv-from-attending-aids-2012-conference. Accessed online September 11th 2012.

Kremer, H., Ironson, G. (2009): Everything Changed: Spiritual Transformation in People with HIV. *The International Journal of Psychiatry in Medicine,* 39: 243-262.

Kremer, H., Ironson, G., Kaplan, L. (2009): The Fork in the Road: HIV as a Potential Positive Turning Point and the Role of Spirituality. *AIDS CARE* 21: 368-377.

Kremer, H., Ironson, G., Schneiderman, N., Hautzinger, M. (2006): To Take or Not to Take: Decision-Making About Antiretroviral Treatment in People Living with HIV/AIDS. *AIDS Patient Care and STDs* 20: 335-349.

Lai, Y.M., Hong, C.P.H., Chee, C.Y.I. (2001): Stigma of Mental Illness. *Singapore Medical Journal,* 42:111-114.

La Veist, T.A. (2002): *Race, Ethnicity, and Health: A Public Health Reader*. California.

LaVeist, T.A., and Amani Nuru-Jeter (2002): Is Doctor-Patient Race Concordance Associated with Greater Satisfaction with Care?" *Journal of Health and Social Behavior,* 43: 296-306.

Lemert, E.M. (1981): Issues in the Study of Deviance." *The Sociological Quarterly,* 22: 285-305.

Lemert, E.M. (1974): Beyond Mead: The Societal Reaction to Deviance. *Social Forces,* 21: 457-468.

Leserman, J., Pettito, J.M., Gu, H., Gaynes, B.N., Barroso, J., Golden, R.N., Perkins, D.O., Folds, J.D., Evans, D.L. (2002): Progression to AIDS, a clinical AIDS condition and mortality: psychosocial and physiological predictors. *Psychological Medicine* 32: 1059-1073.

Leserman, J., Pettito, J.M., Golden, R.N., Gaynes, B.N., Gu, H., Perkins, D.O., Silva, S.G., Folds, J.D., Evans, D.L. (2000): Impact of Stressful Life Events, Depression, Social Support, Coping, and Cortisol on Progression to AIDS. *American Journal of Psychiatry,* 157: 1221-1228.

Link, B.G., Castille, D.M., Stuber, J. (2008): Stigma and coercion in the context of outpatient treatment for people with mental illnesses. *Social Science and Medicine,* 67: 409-419.

Link, B.G., Phelan, J.C. (2006): Stigma and its Public Health Implications. *The Lancet,* 367: 528-529.

Link, B.G., Phelan, J.C. (2001): Conceptualizing Stigma. *Annual Review of Sociology,* 27: 363-385.

Link B.G., Phelan, J.C., Bresnahan, M., Stueve, A., Pescosolido, B.A. (1999): Public Conceptions of Mental Illness: Labels, Causes, Dangerousness, and Social Distance. *American Journal of Public Health,* 89:1328-1333.

Link, B.G., Struening, E.L., Rahav, M., Phelan, J.C., Nuttbrock, L. (1997): On Stigma and its Consequences: Evidence from a Longitudinal Study of Men with Dual Diagnoses of Mental Illness and Substance Abuse. *Journal of Health and Social Behavior,* 38: 177-190.

Link, B.G., Cullen, F.T., Struening, E., Shrout, P.E., Dohrenwend, B.P. (1989): A Modified Labeling Theory Approach to Mental Disorders: An Empirical Assessment. *American Sociological Review* 54: 400-423.

Lichtenstein, B., Hook III, E.W., Sharma, A.K. (2005): Public Tolerance, Private Pain: Stigma and Sexually Transmitted Infections in the American Deep South. *Culture, Health and Sexuality*, 7: 43-57.

Liu, H., Feng, T., Ha, T., Liu, H., Cai, Y. (2006): Chinese Culture, Homosexuality stigma, Social Support and Condom Use: A Path Analytic Model. *Stigma Research and Action*, 1:27-35.

Lutz, F., Kremer, H., Ironson, G. (2011): Being Diagnosed with HIV as a Trigger for Spiritual Transformation. *Religions* 2: 398-409.

Mahajan, A.P., Sayles, J.N., Patel, V.A., Remien, R.H., Ortiz, D., Szekeres, G., Coates, T.J. (2008): Stigma in the HIV/AIDS Epidemic: A review of the literature and recommnedations for the way forward. *AIDS* 22:67-79.

Mann, J. (1987): Statement at an informal briefing on AIDS to the 42nd Session of the United Nations General Assembly, 20 October, New York.

Markowitz, F.E. (1998): The Effects of Stigma on the Psychological Well-Being and Life Satis- faction of Persons with Mental Illness. *Journal of Health and Social Behavior*, 39: 335-347.

Massey, S., Cameron, A., Ouellette, S., Fine, M. (1998): Qualitative Approaches to the Study of Thriving: What Can Be Leanred? *Journal of Social Issues*, 54: 337-355.

Massey, D.S., Denton, N.A. (1993): *American Apartheid: Segregation and the Making of the Underclass*. Cambridge.

McCann, L., Illingworth, N., Wengstrom, Y., Hubbard, G., Kearney, N. (2010): Transitional experiences of women with breast cancer within the first year following diagnosis. *Journal of Clinical Nursing*, 19, 1969-1976.

McEwen, B. (2002): *The end of stress as we know it*. Washington DC.

McLeod, J.D., Shanahan, M.J. (1996): Trajectories of poverty and children's mental health. *Journal of Health and Social Behavior*, 37: 207-220.

Mead, G.H. (1934): *Mind, Self, and Society: From the Standpoint of a Social Behaviorist*. Chicago.

Medley, A.M., Kennedy, C.E., Lunyolo, S., Sweat, M.D. (2009): Disclosure Outcomes, Coping Strategies, and Life Changes Among Women Living with HIV in Uganda. *Qualitative Health Research* 19: 1744-1754.

Merton, R.K. (1968): *Social Theory and Social Structure*. New York.

Merton, R.K. (1957): The Role-Set: Problems in Sociological Theory. *The British Journal of Sociology*, 8: 106-120.

Merton, R.K. (1938): Social Structure and Anomie. *American Sociological Review*, 3: 672-682.

Messner, S.F., Rosenfeld, R. (2007): *Crime and the American Dream*. 4th ed., Monterey.

Michels, I.I., Stöver, H., Gerlach, R. (2007): Subsitution Treatment for Opioid Addicts in Germany. *Harm Reduction Journal*, 4: 1477-7517.

Miech, R.A., Caspi, A., Moffitt, T.E., Entner Wright, B.R., Silva, P.A. (1999): Low Socioeconomic Status and Mental Disorders: A Longitudinal Study of Selection and Causation During Young Adulthood. *The American Journal of Sociology*, 104: 1096-1131.

Milam, J. (2006): Posttraumatic Growth and HIV Disease Progression. *Journal of Consulting and Clinical Psychology*, 74: 817-827.

Milloy, M.-J. S., Marshall, B.D.L., Kerr, T., Buxton, J., Rhodes, T., Montaner, J., Wood, E. (2012): Social and structural factors associated with HIV disease progression among illicit drug users: a systematic review. *AIDS*, 26:1049-1063.

Mossakowski, K.N., Kaplan, L.M., Hill, T.D. (2011): Americans' Attitudes toward Mental Illness and Involuntary Psychiatric Medication. *Society and Mental Health*, 1: 200-216.

Mulder, C.L., Antoni, M.H., Duivenvoorden, H.J., Kauffmann, R.H., Goodkin, K. (1995): Active Confrontational Coping Predicts Decreased Clinical Progression Over a One-Year Period in HIV-Infected Homosexual Men. *Journal of Psychosomatic Research* 39: 957-965.

Norredam, M., Mygind, A., Krasnik, A. (2005): Access to Health Care for Asylum Seekers in the European Union – A Comparative Study of Country Policies. *European Journal of Public Health*, Advanced Access published October 17, 2005.

OECD (2012a): OECD Economic Surveys: Germany 2012, OECD Publishing.

OECD (2012b): OECD Economic Surveys: United States 2012, OECD Publishing.

OECD (2012c): Income Inequality in the European Union: Economics Department Working Papers no. 952, OECD Publishing.

O'Leary, V.E. (1998): Strength in the Face of Adversity: Individual and Social Thriving. *Journal of Social Issues,* 54: 425-446.

O'Leary. V.E., Ickovics, J.R. (1995): Resilience and Thriving in Response to Challenge: An Opportunity for a Paradigm Shift in Women's Health. *Women's Health: Research on Gender. Behavior, and Policy,* 1: 121- 142.

Ogunmefun, C., Gilbert, L., Schatz, E. (2011): Older Female Caregivers and HIV/AIDS-Related Secondary Stigma in Rural South Africa. *Journal of Cross Cultural Gerontology,* 26: 85-102.

Oman, D. (2010): Compassionate Love: What Does the Research Show? Report to Fetzer Institute. Revised 3rd version: September 9, 2010.

Parker, R., Aggleton, P., Attawell, K., Pulerwitz, J., Brown, L. (2002): HIV/AIDS-Related Stigma and Discrimination: A Conceptual Framework and an Agenda for Action. Population Council Report. Accessed online: August 1st, 2012.

Parker, R., Aggleton, P. (2003): HIV and AIDS-related Stigma and Discrimination: A conceptual Framework and Implications for Action. *Social Science and Medicine,* 57: 13-24.

Pearlin, L.I., Schieman, S., Fazio, E.M., Meersman, S.C. (2005): Stress, Health, and the Life Course: Some Conceptual Perspectives. *Journal of Health and Social Behavior* 46: 205-219.

Pearlin, L.I. (1989): The Sociological Study of Stress. *Journal of Health and Social Behavior,* 30: 241-256.

Pearlin, L.I., Menaghan, E.G., Lieberman, M.A., Mullan, J.T. (1981): The Stress Process. *Journal of Health and Social Behavior,* 22: 337-356.

Perleberg, K., Schütze, F., Heine, V. (2006): Sozialwissenschaftliche Biographieanalyse von chronisch kranken Patientinnen auf der empirischen Grundlage des autobiographisch-narrativen Interviews. *Psychotherapie und Sozialwissenschaft* 1/2006, S. 95-145.

Pescosolido, B.A., Monahan, J., Link, B.G., Stueve, A., Kikuzawa, S. (1999): The Public's View of the Competence, Dangerousness, and Need for Legal Coercion of Persons with Mental Health Problems. *American Journal of Public Health,* 89:1339-345.

Pew Research Center (2012): The Rise of Residential Segregation by Income. *Pew Social and Demographic Trends.* Wednesday, August 1, 2012. Washington DC.

Pierret, J. (2001): Interviews and Biographical Time: The Case of Long-Term HIV Nonprogressors. *Sociology of Health and Illness,* 23: 157-179.

Primomo, J., Yates, B.C., Woods, N.F. (1990): Social Support for Women During Chronic Illness: The Relationship between Sources and Types of Adjustment. *Research and Nursing Health* 13: 153-161.

Reuters (2013): EU Leaders Rebuff Calls for Action on Europe's Migration Crisis. http://www.reuters.com/article/2013/10/25/us-eu-migrants-idUSBRE99O0NB20131025. Accessed December 18th, 2013.

Riemann, G., Schütze, F. (1991): Trajectory" as a Basic Theoretical Concept for Analyzing Suffering and Disorderly Social Processes. In: David, R. (ed.): *Social Organization and Social Processes.* Essays In Honor of Anselm Strauss. Hawthorne, N.Y., pp. 333-347.

Riemann, G. (2003): A Joint Project Against the Backdrop of a Research Tradition: An Introduction to "Doing Biographical Research" [36 paragraphs]. *Forum Qualitative Sozialforschung / Forum: Qualitative Social Research 4* (3) 2003. www.qualitative research.net/index.php/fqs/article/view/666/1440. [Accessed December 18th, 2008].

Ross, M.W., Berg, R.C., Schmidt, A.J., Hospers, H.J., Breveglieri, M., Furegato, M., Weatherburn, P. (2013); Internalised homonegativity predicts HIV-associated risk behavior in European men who have sex with men in a 38-country cross-sectional study: some public health implications of homophobia. *BMJ Open.* 3.doi:10.1136/bmjopen-2012-001928. Downloaded from bmjopen.bmj.com on February 5, 2013.

Ross, M.W.E., Essien, J., Torres, I. (2006): Conspiracy Beliefs about the Origin of HIV/AIDS in Four Racial/Ethnic Groups. *Journal of Acquired Immune Deficiency Syndromes,* 41: 342-344.

Sacks, H. (1967): The Search for Help: No one to Turn to. In: E.S. Schneidman (ed.): *Essays in Self Destruction.* New York, NY, pp. 203-233.

Safren, S.A., Gershuny, B.S., Hendriksen, E. (2003): Symptoms of Posttraumatic Stress and Death Anxiety in Persons with HIV and Medication Adherence Difficulties. *AIDS Patient Care and STDs,* 17: 657-664.

Salter, M.L., Go, V.F., Minh, N.L., Gregowski, A., Ha, T.V., Rudolph, A., Latkin, C., Celentano, D.D., Quan, V.M. (2010): Influence of Perceived Secondary Stigma and Family on the Response to HIV infection Among Injection Drug Users in Vietnam. *AIDS Education and Prevention,* 22: 558-570.

Sandstrom, K.L. (1996): Redefining Sex and Intimacy: The Sexual Self-Images, Outlooks, and Relationships of Gay Men Living with HIV/AIDS. *Symbolic Interaction,* 3: 241-262.

Scambler, G. (2004): Re-framing Stigma: Felt and Enacted Stigma and Challenges to the Sociology of Chronic and Disabling Conditions. *Social Theory and Health,* 2: 29-46.

Scandlyn, Jean (2000): When AIDS became a Chronic Disease. *The Western Journal of Medicine,* 172: 130-133.

Scheff, T.J. (1990): *Microsociology: Discourse, Emotion, and Social Structure.* Chicago.

Shinn, M., Lehmann, S.. Wong, N.W. (1984): Social Interaction and Social Support. *Society for the Psychological Study of Social Issues* 55-76.

Schütz, A. (1962): *Collected Papers: I The Problem of Social Reality.* The Hague.

Schütze, F., Schröder-Wildhagen, A., Inowlocki, L., Nagel, U., Riemann, G., Treichel, B. (2010): Discoverers in the European Mental Space – The Biographical Experiences of Participants in European Civil Society Organizations. Working Paper.

Schütze, F. (2007): Biography analysis on the empirical base of autobiographical narratives: How to analyse autobiographical narrative interviews – part I. Module B.2.1. *INVITE – Biographical counselling in rehabilitative vocational training – further education curriculum.* Verfügbar über: www.biographicalcounselling.com/download/B2.1.pdf [Accessed online 10.01.2013].

Schütze, F. (2005): Eine sehr persönlich generalisierte Sicht auf qualitative Forschung. *Zeitschrift für qualitative Bildungs-, Beratungs- und Sozialforschung. ZBBS* 6. Jg., Heft 2/2005, S. 211-248.

Schütze, F. (2001): Rätselhafte Stellen im narrativen Interview. Handlung Kultur Interpretation, Jg. 10, Heft 1, S.12-28.

Schütze, F. (1992): Pressure and guilt. War experiences of a young German soldier and their biographical implications. *International Sociology,* 7: 187-208; 7(3), 347-367.

Schütze, F. (1984): Kognitive Figuren des autobiographischen Stegreiferzählens. In: Kohli, M., Robert, G. (eds.): *Biographie und soziale Wirklichkeit.* Neue Beiträge und Forschungsperspek- tiven, Stuttgart, S. 78- 117.

Schütze, F. (1981): Prozessstrukturen des Lebensablaufs. In: Matthes, J., Pfeifenberger, A., Stosberg, M. (eds.): *Biographie in handlungswissenschaftlicher Perspektive.* Nürnberg, pp. 67-156.

Schütze, F. (1983): Biographieforschung und narratives Interview. *Neue Praxis* 3, 283-293.

Schwenk A., Breuer, J.P., Kremer, G., Römer, K., Bethe, U., Franzen, C., Fätkenheuer, G., Salzberger, B. (2000): Risk factors for the HIV-associated lipodystrophy syndrome in a cross- sectional single-centre study. *European Journal of Medical Research* 5:443-448.

Scollay, P.A., Doucett, M., Perry, M., Winterbottom, B. (1992): AIDS education of college students: The effect of an HIV-positive lecturer. *AIDS Education and Prevention,* 4: 160-171.

Siebert, H. (2003): Germany: An immigration country. Kiel Working Papers, No. 1189, http://hdl.handle.net/10419/3099.

Siegel, K., Schrimshaw, E.W. (2000): Perceiving benefits in adversity: stress-related growth in women living with HIV/AIDS. *Social Science and Medicine* 51: 1543-1554.

Siegel, K., Krauss, B.J. (1991): Living with HIV Infection: Adaptive Tasks of Seropositive Gay Men. *Journal of Health and Social Behavior,* 32: 17-32.

Smart, L., Wegner, D.M. (1999): Covering Up What Can't Be Seen: Concealable Stigma and Mental Control. *Journal of Personality and Social Psychology* 77: 474-486.

Smit, P.J., Brady, M., Carter, M., Fernandes, R., Lamore, L., Meulbroek, M., Ohayon, M., Platteau, T., Rehberg, P., Rockstroh, J.K., Thompson, M. (2011): AIDS Care: Psychological and Socio-medical Aspects of AIDS/HIV. *AIDS Care,* 24: 405-412.

Solano, L., Costa, M., Temoshok, L., Salvati, S., Coda, R., Aiuti, F. (2002): An Emotionally Inexpressive (Type C) Coping Style Influences HIV Disease Progression at Six and Twelve Month Follow-Ups. *Psychology and Health* 17:641-655.

Sorokin, P.A. (1954, 2002): *The ways and power of love: Types, factors, and techniques of moral transformation.* Philadelphia.

Stangor, C., Crandall, C.S. (2000): Threat and the social construction of stigma. In: Heatherton, T.F., Kleck, R.E., Hebl, M.R., Hull, J.G. (eds.): *The social psychology of stigma.* New York, pp. 62-87.

Steele, C.M., Aronson, J. (1995): Stereotype Threat and Intellectual Test Performance of African Americans. *Journal of Personality and Social Psychology* 69: 797-811.

Strauss, A.L. (1997): *Mirrors and Masks: The Search for Identity.* New Jersey.

Strauss, A.L., Faherhaugh, S., Suczek, B. (1997): *Social Organization of Medical Work.* New Jersey.

Strauss, A.L. (1993): *Continual Permutations of Action.* New York.

Stryker, S. (1980): *Symbolic Interactionism: A Social Structural Version.* Palto Alto.

Tajfel, H., Turner, J. (1986): The Social Identity Theory of Group Behavior. In: Worchel, S., Austin, W.G. (eds.): *Psychology of Intergroup Relations..* Chicago, pp. 7-24.

The Brookings Institution (2004): *The Rise of New Immigrant Gateways.* The Living Cities Census Series. Washington, DC.

The Guardian (2013): 'Hartz Reforms': How a Benefits Shakeup Changed Germany. http://www.theguardian.com/commentisfree/2013/jan/01/germany-hartz-reforms-inequality. Accessed online September, 4th 2013.

The Local (2012): 'Immigrants Cause Problems' Say Germans. Published: 17 Dec 12 12:39 CET. Accessed online February, 7th 2013.

The World Conference on Human Rights (1993): Vienna Declaration and Programme of Action. June 25th 1993. Vienna, Austria.

Thoits, P. (1995): Stress, Coping, and Social Support, Processes: Where Are We? What Next? *Journal of Health and Social Behavior,* 35: 53-79.

Thomas, W.I., Znaniecki, F. (1927): *The Polish Peasant in Europe.* New York, NY.

Torian, L.V., Wiewel, E.W. (2011): Continuity of HIV-Related Medical Care, New York City, 2005–2009: Do Patients Who Initiate Care Stay in Care?*AIDS PATIENT CARE and STDs,* 25: 79-88.

Turner, R.J., Wheaton, B.L. (1995): The Epidemiology of Social Stress. *American Sociological Review,* 60: 104-125.

UNAIDS (2012): *Global AIDS Response Country Progress Report: Germany.* http://www.unaids.org/en/dataanalysis/knowyourresponse/countryprogressreports/2012countries/ce_DE_Narrative_Report[1].pdf. Accessed online January 28, 2013.

UNAIDS (2005): *HIV-Related Stigma, Discrimination and Human Rights Violations.* UNAIDS Best Practice Collection.

UNAIDS (2008): *Report on the Global AIDS Epidemic.* Geneva, UNAIDS.

UNAIDS (2009): *AIDS Epidemic Update: November 2009.* Geneva, UNAIDS.

United Nations, Economic and Social Council. Committee on Economic, Social, and Cultural Rights (2012): *Report on the Forty-Six and Forty-Seventh Sessions.* New York.

United Nations, Department of Economic and Social Affairs (2005): *Population, Development and HIV/AIDS with Particular Emphasis on Poverty: The Concise Report.* New York.

Underwood, L.G. (2008): Compassionate Love: A Framework for Research. In: Fehr, B., Sprecher, S., Underwood, L.G. (eds.): *The Science of Compassionate Love: Theory, Research, and Applications.* Malden, MA, pp. 3-25.

U.S. Census Bureau (2013): *State and County QuickFacts*. Data derived from Population Estimates, American Community Survey, Census of Population and Housing, State and County Housing Unit Estimates, County Business Patterns, Nonemployer Statistics, Economic Census, Survey of Business Owners, Building Permits, Consolidated Federal Funds Report. Last Revised: Thursday, 10-Jan-2013 15:08:12 EST.

Weber, M. (1930): *The Protestant Ethic and the Spirit of Capitalism*. (Translated by Talcott Parsons and Anthony Giddens). London and Boston.

Weber, M. (1949): *The Methodology of the Social Sciences*. Editor: E.A.. Shils. Translated by H.A. Finch. New York.

Weber, M. (1978): *Economy and Society: An Outline of Interpretive Sociology*. Editors: G. Roth, C. Wittich. Berkeley.

Weinold, M., Ramazan, S., Ngassa Djomo, K. (2007): *Germany Country Report: EU Partnerships to reduce HIV and public health vulnerabilities associated with population mobility.* http://www.iom.int/jahia/webdav/shared/shared/mainsite/activities/health/eu_ consultation/country_report_germany.pdf. Accessed online January 28, 2013.

Williams, G. (1984): The Genesis of Chronic Illness: Narrative Re-Construction. *Sociology of Health and Illness,* 6: 176-200.

Williams, D.R., Collins, C. (1995): US Socioeconomic and Racial Differences in Health: Patterns and Explanations. *Annual Review of Sociology,* 21: 349-86.

Wilson, S. (2007): 'When you have children, you're obliged to live': motherhood, chronic illness, and biographical disruption. *Sociology of Health and Illness,* 29: 610-626.

World Health Organization (1948): *Preamble to the Constitution of the World Health Organization as adopted by the International Health Conference.* New York, 19-22 June, 1946; signed on 22 July 1946 by the representatives of 61 States (Official Records of the World Health Organization, no. 2, p. 100) and entered into force on 7 April 1948.